Praise for *Smart Fat*

"Perhaps the most damaging but still pervasive notion in healthy nutrition has been the castigation of fat. *Smart Fat* provides an eloquent foundation for the critical health-supportive attributes of fat in the human diet. This wonderful book paves the way to welcome this critical nutrient back to the table, opening the door for health and disease resistance."

> —David Perlmutter, M.D., F.A.C.N., board-certified neurologist and
> *New York Times* bestselling author of *Grain Brain* and *Brain Maker*

"*Smart Fat* is a groundbreaking book that's going to create a seismic shift in how we look at fat *and* why we need much more of it in our diet. A must-read!"

> —JJ Virgin, *New York Times* bestselling author of *Sugar Impact Diet*

"*Smart Fat* perfectly illustrates what I tell my clients and readers: It's not about calories, it's about eating foods that are hormonally helpful; it's not about eating less or more, it's about eating smarter. This is a smart book by two of the smartest experts in the field."

> —Sara Gottfried, M.D., *New York Times* bestselling author
> of *The Hormone Reset Diet*

"*Smart Fat* is written brilliantly, filled to the brim with the research necessary to back up the authors' claims and destined to become a nutritional classic. I love both these men's astute minds and know the passion that they both share with their work. Having them join forces to write a book is a dream come true!"

> —Leanne Ely, C.N.C., *New York Times* bestselling author
> and the founder of SavingDinner.com

"*Smart Fat* spells out a simple new understanding of which fats can improve your health and which will set you back. By learning which fats are good, which are bad, and which are neutral, you can easily shed unwanted weight and cut the risk of heart disease and other chronic diseases."

> —Alan Christianson, N.M.D., *New York Times* bestselling author
> of *The Adrenal Reset Diet* and founder of Integrative Health

"The non-fat-diet craze years ago created many health problems for people, including increasing the obesity rates. The solution has not been to cut down on fat but instead to learn about the importance of healthy fats. Once again Dr. Masley and Dr. Bowden have mastered getting out the information in a simple, comprehensive way that is guaranteed to make changes for the better of your health. Wonderful ideas and great menus. Nicely done."

—Marcelle Pick, ob-gyn and pediatric nurse practitioner, founder
of WomentoWomen.com and author of *The Core Balance Diet,
Is It Me or My Adrenals?,* and *Is It Me or My Hormones?*

"*Smart Fat* comes to us at a critical time. It is easy to read, easy to implement, and will definitely help your brain work better so you can too."

—Daniel G. Amen, M.D., founder of Amen Clinics and author
of *Change Your Brain, Change Your Life*

"Do you want gorgeous skin, glowing health, balanced hormones, a slim body, and amazing energy? Then stop listening to out-of-date doctors who tell you to shun fat and start reading *Smart Fat*. And do it right now—because this revolutionary book will change your life, and it may even save it."

—Kellyann Petrucci, N.M.D., author of *Dr. Kellyann's Bone Broth Diet* and
creator of the public television special "21 Days to a Younger, Slimmer You"

"Recent scientific investigations have determined that almost half of the U.S. population is pre-diabetic as well as overtly diabetic. The fix is easy with simple lifestyle solutions that absolutely work. Drs. Masley and Bowden have outlined a strategic plan in *Smart Fat* and offer the reader many creative options to dismantle insulin resistance, diabetes, and metabolic syndrome."

—Stephen T. Sinatra, M.D., F.A.C.N., cardiologist and coauthor
of *Health Revelations from Heaven and Earth*

"Finally, a book that helps eliminate our irrational fear of fat! Steven Masley and Jonny Bowden break through one of our most ingrained beliefs about food. They skillfully replace fear and with fiercely smart strategies for nourishing your body, brain, and overall health."

—Dr. Susan Albers, psychologist and *New York Times* bestselling author of
EatQ, Eating Mindfully, and *50 Ways to Soothe Yourself Without Food*

SMART FAT

SMART FAT

Eat More Fat.
Lose More Weight.
Get Healthy Now.

Steven Masley, M.D.
and **Jonny Bowden, Ph.D., C.N.S.**

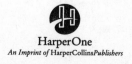

HarperOne
An Imprint of HarperCollins*Publishers*

HarperOne

SMART FAT. Copyright © 2016 by Jonny Bowden and Steven Masley, M.D. All rights reserved. Printed in the United States of America. No part of this book may be used or reproduced in any manner whatsoever without written permission except in the case of brief quotations embodied in critical articles and reviews. For information address HarperCollins Publishers, 195 Broadway, New York, NY 10007.

HarperCollins books may be purchased for educational, business, or sales promotional use. For information please e-mail the Special Markets Department at SPsales@harpercollins.com.

HarperCollins website: http://www.harpercollins.com

FIRST EDITION

Designed by Terry McGrath

Library of Congress Cataloging-in-Publication Data
Bowden, Jonny, author.
Smart fat : eat more fat, lose more weight, get healthy now / Jonny Bowden, Ph.D., C.N.S. and Steven Masley, M.D. —First edition.
    pages cm
Includes index.
ISBN 978–0–06–239229–9
1. Weight loss. 2. Essential fatty acids in human nutrition.
3. Food preferences. 4. Self-care, Health. I. Masley, Steven. II. Title.
RM222.2B6465 2016
613.2'5—dc23

                            2015015983

15 16 17 18 19   RRD(H)   10 9 8 7 6 5 4 3 2 1

*This book is dedicated to my many patients for sharing
their true struggles—their triumphs remain my
inspiration and their encouragement my motivation.*
—Steven Masley

To the memory of Elliot and Vivienne Bowden.
—Jonny Bowden

Contents

INTRODUCTION   The Smartest Way to Live for the Rest of Your Life   1

PART ONE—SMART FACTS ABOUT SMART FAT

CHAPTER 1   A High-Fat Diet for a Low-Fat Body   9

CHAPTER 2   Why the Smart Fat Solution Will Make You Lean and Healthy   17

CHAPTER 3   What *Not* to Eat   46

CHAPTER 4   Unlearn What You Know About Food   68

PART TWO—SMART-FAT YOUR FOOD

CHAPTER 5   The Smart Fat Solution   97

CHAPTER 6   The Thirty-Day Plan of Smart Fat Meals   119

CHAPTER 7   The Smart Fat User's Guide   136

PART THREE—BEYOND DIET: SMART FOR LIFE

CHAPTER 8   Smart Supplements   169

CHAPTER 9   Smart Living   197

CHAPTER 10   Smart Recipes   220

REFERENCES   285

ACKNOWLEDGMENTS   301

RECIPE INDEX   305

SUBJECT INDEX   315

The Smartest Way to Live
for the Rest of Your Life

THERE IS A WAY OF EATING that will change your life forever.

You *will* lose weight, and keep it off.

You *will* feel and look better than ever.

You *will* get—and stay—healthy.

We're confident that you've never tried to eat like this before, because up until now, the advice on what to eat (and what to avoid) has been difficult to follow. Should you eat low-carb? Low-fat? Paleo? Raw food? Vegan? High-protein? And what about high-fiber?

All of these dietary approaches have their legions of die-hard followers and sworn supporters, from respected medical and science professionals and fitness gurus, to celebrity endorsers touting their before-and-after photos. There are dozens of best-selling books on all these topics, huge amounts of constantly changing information and research, and countless online resources—all of which any of us can access at any time.

A lot of information is out there, which makes for a great deal of confusion, because none of it ever seems to answer your question: *What should I eat to lose weight and be healthy?*

One of us (Jonny) is a well-known nutritionist and author, a renowned expert on weight loss and wellness who has helped thousands of people reach their goals and get healthy. The other (Steven) is a highly respected physician, nutritionist, author, and patient educator who has devoted much of his career to the study of heart disease and aging, publishing research on these topics in major medical journals.

We independently came to the same conclusion about why so many people fail, over and over again, to lose weight and get healthy. We'll fill in the rest of this story in the chapters to come, but here's the point: Despite current popular opinion, fat is a critical component of your health. When we decided to banish fat from our diets, we lost its considerable health benefits.

In fact, eating *more fat* is the best way to achieve optimal health, longevity, and permanent weight loss.

But, before you get too excited and start loading up on butter and oil, let's be clear about our message. The high-fat diet we're recommending will make you healthier and slim for life, but only if you do two things: First, you've got to eat lots of what we call "smart fat." Second, you have to consume smart fat with the right amounts of fiber and protein, all of which have to be infused with great flavor. As you'll see, the herbs and spices that season our food not only have major health benefits, they are also the reason why you'll enjoy eating this way for the rest of your life.

If you're wondering about what kind of food and how much of it to eat, rest assured that we'll tell you. But first, let's talk about fat.

The problem is not the *amount* of fat in our diets, as we were led to believe for many decades. The problem is that in the name of good health, we mistakenly stripped out of our meals, our kitchens, our restaurants, and our grocery stores the beneficial *smart fat*—healthy, natural dietary fat from clean, wholesome sources. We replaced it with low-fat (and fat-free) "healthy" food, which turned out to be anything *but* healthy. Not only were these foodlike products low in beneficial fats, they were high in processed carbohydrates and sugar, which are *very* bad for our brains, hearts, and waistlines.

To make matters worse, although we encouraged people to keep some fats on the table, we promoted the wrong kinds of fats. These not-so-smart-fats (go ahead—call them *dumb fats*) found in prepared and processed foods, and in animal products produced in crowded factories, were precisely the worst fats for health (and for weight loss), but they've infiltrated our diet at our own invitation, and they continue to do plenty of damage to this day.

But we now know, after years of research and extensive studies, that healthy dietary fat should *not* be avoided, that we should, in fact, eat *more* smart fats. And in the following pages we're going to show you how to do just that—the right way.

We're hardly alone in saying that fat is essential for our health and well-being. Since 2010, a spate of studies have come out vindicating fat—even saturated fat—of any direct role in heart disease. But unfortunately, when the "it's okay to eat fat!" news jumped from medical journals and into the daily newsfeed, a key question frequently went unanswered: *What kind of fat should we incorporate into our diets?*

That's one of the important questions about health that this book answers for you.

We've been so concerned with "saturated vs. unsaturated" and "animal vs. vegetable" that we've lost sight of a far more important distinction: *toxic vs. nontoxic fat*—or, as we call it, dumb fat vs. smart fat. There are some critical health- and weight-related reasons why this distinction is so crucial, and you'll be hearing a lot more about them in the chapters that follow.

As you're about to see, eating a cheeseburger and fries, digging into a plate of fettuccine Alfredo, snacking on a donut, or downing a root beer float is not the take-away from the latest science, but we'll tell you what *is*. We're here to clear up the confusion about what kind of fat to eat, and we're *also* here to give you a plan: the Smart Fat Solution.

We've found a path to healthy weight loss and a lifetime of wellness, and it's surprisingly simple to follow. Your challenge is making the decision to *take* this path, to think a bit differently about your daily diet, and to accept that this new way of eating will transform your life—for the better.

It all comes down to this: If you want the same results, keep doing the same thing you're doing now. Keep eating the same way, keep living the same way. And you know what? You're likely to get more of the same. You won't lose any weight, and you'll probably gain more. You won't feel any better, and you won't have any more energy. But why would you? Eating the way you've been eating hasn't worked so far, so why would it suddenly start producing a healthier, fitter, happier you?

We know, that sounds like tough love—because it is. But without the truth, you can't do anything to make things better. And we want to show you *how* to make things better.

You're about to *unlearn* what you know about fat, and in the process you'll find the ideal weight-loss and eating plan that you can follow for a lifetime of vibrant, good health. That's the Smart Fat Solution. You'll love how you feel (and how you look), and you're going to enjoy the flavors of great ingredients that are a pleasure to prepare and eat. And, we predict, you'll wonder why you never approached food this way in the first place, particularly if you've bounced from diet to diet without success.

If you're *really* looking for genuine, lasting change in how you look and how you feel—if you want different, *better* results—then it's time to do things differently.

In the following pages, you'll find life-changing information about the vital role that smart fat (nutritional fat) plays in our well-being and longevity. You'll also find information about what most people incorrectly think of as "good" fat.

Medically sound, scientifically based—and best of all—user-friendly, the Smart Fat Solution is designed so that you can follow it for the rest of your life. Once you get started, you'll

- Lose unwanted weight and keep it off—and lower your body fat
- Feel more energetic and healthier than ever
- Manage stress better
- Have improved brain function
- Dramatically reduce accelerated aging of the body and brain
- Prevent and even reverse heart disease and type 2 diabetes
- Decrease your risk for developing cancer and other life-threatening illnesses
- Lower your susceptibility to nagging chronic conditions

It's time to get smart about fat—and about everything else that goes into feeling your very best.

Jonny and Steven

PART ONE

Smart Facts About Smart Fat

CHAPTER 1

A High-Fat Diet
for a Low-Fat Body

NOT TOO LONG AGO, we both were advocating specific diets for
weight loss and wellness. We weren't just advocates of these
plans—we built our professional lives around these two seemingly
contradictory nutritional philosophies.

As a practicing nutritionist, Jonny championed the ultra-low-carb
Atkins Diet. Famous for its high-protein intake and its jump-start
approach to weight loss, Atkins let people lose weight quickly, especially individuals with a lot of excess pounds to shed. But despite the
diet's short-term success, Jonny was troubled by its sometimes restrictive approach, as well as some of the highly processed foods on the
diet's "okay to eat" list, specifically deli meats, which were liberally
allowed.

His instinct was to add more variety, including additional plant
sources of fiber such as beans and legumes, which are also great
sources of protein, as well as low-sugar fruits like berries. Jonny preferred "clean" protein instead of the protein from processed, commercial animal products such as feedlot farmed meat and processed

cheeses, all of which can be contaminated with additives, hormones, and pesticides. But these modifications didn't always adhere to the rigid parameters of the Atkins Diet.

Meanwhile, Steven—a physician, nutritionist, trained chef, and medical fellow with several prestigious health organizations—held the position of medical director at the Pritikin Longevity Center where he oversaw many aspects of healthy weight loss, including the center's ultra-low-fat eating plan. Pritikin participants often struggled with serious conditions like life-threatening heart disease and diabetes. After their stay at Pritikin—with its carefully regulated diet of whole, unprocessed foods high in fiber and complex carbohydrates—people would lose weight quickly, drop several of their medications, and leave the center in excellent shape.

But Steven noticed a troubling pattern: After participants left the controlled surroundings of the Pritikin Center, they regularly returned to their old ways. They just couldn't stick with the program on their own. Steven, who has spent years researching cardiac health and observing thousands of patients, knew that the Pritikin Diet lacked the healthy proteins and important fats that would have rounded out a truly nutritious and effective diet that a person could follow for life. But just as Jonny found out trying to experiment with the Atkins Diet, any kind of variety or modification, no matter how healthy, wasn't allowed within the strictly regimented protocol of the Pritikin Diet.

Though thousands of miles apart on different coasts of the United States, we independently came to the same conclusion: Both the Atkins and Pritikin diets—and the countless other popular diets that millions of Americans follow—were missing the critical components for long-term success. They were hard to sustain, and almost impossible to adopt as a daily way of eating. Yes, they promised impressive short-term results, but neither diet offered any long-term, sustainable results. Neither Atkins nor Pritikin, we realized, was enough to help people lose weight, keep it off, and remain healthy for the rest of their lives.

The Atkins Diet, for instance, featured foods with ample amounts of protein and fat, while limiting foods with refined carbohydrates in order to keep the glycemic load low. (We'll explain later why properly identifying refined carbs and glycemic *load*—not glycemic *index*—is crucial to your success.) But the diet was deficient in fiber and certain nutrients, such as anti-aging plant pigments like carotenoids and flavonoids, and disease-fighting vitamins and minerals, including vitamins C and K, as well as magnesium and potassium. These are all necessary for optimal health. Atkins also featured foods with potentially high amounts of factory-farmed beef, pork, and poultry and mass-produced dairy products—all of which are likely to be contaminated with toxic hormones, pesticides, and chemicals.

Though neither plan was ideal, they were still vast improvements over the way most Americans were eating by the 1970s. By then, we were wrongly blaming fat for all our health woes, from heart disease to cancer. The Pritikin and Atkins diets, as well as many other well-known weight-loss programs, were finding a ready audience among increasing numbers of people who were desperate to lose weight and regain their health. Though the dietary "solutions" to this crisis varied dramatically, the crisis was caused by one problem: the Standard American Diet (or, fittingly, SAD), which took hold after we banished healthy smart fats.

The SAD actually featured the worst of Atkins (processed protein) and the worst of Pritikin (insufficient healthy fats and protein), combined with a heaping side of refined carbohydrates and processed convenience foods, prepared with so-called heart-healthy "vegetable" oils and deadly, artificial trans fats, used in shelf-stable convenience foods and fast foods. A day's eating might include sugary cereal, toast slathered with trans fat–packed margarine, and juice for breakfast; a sandwich of processed deli meats for lunch (plus fries or chips and a package of cookies for dessert); more processed meat for dinner (or frozen fish sticks)—and maybe, just maybe, a tiny portion of vegetables, like ketchup.

Another starring component of the SAD besides processed foods and dumb fats was sugar—lots and lots of sugar, in many different forms and from many different sources: from the usual suspects like candy, soda, and artificially sweetened drinks, and from packaged cookies, crackers, pretzels, chips, muffins, and other commercially manufactured baked goods—many of them made with high-fructose corn syrup. But these were just the obvious ones. The very basis of the SAD was large servings of starchy carbohydrates that quickly *convert* to sugar in the body—foods like pasta, white rice and bread, and "healthy" items like sweetened fat-free yogurt and granola bars. From your body's point of view, you might as well have swallowed the entire sugar bowl.

Now, after decades of the SAD, and fruitlessly searching for magic-bullet diets that we can use to eat ourselves out of being sicker and fatter, here is what we've wrought:

- Heart disease is still the No. 1 killer in our country, claiming more than six hundred thousand lives a year in the United States.
- Fifty-nine percent of Americans are actively trying to lose weight every year, but only 5 to 10 percent manage to keep weight off. More than a third of our population is obese.
- Diabetes and its many complications have ruined the lives of millions, including children.
- Metabolic Syndrome, or prediabetes—a lethal combination of risk factors for heart disease and diabetes (which we'll explore in detail in Chapter 4)—is on track to become the Black Plague of the twenty-first century. One out of three people have it.
- Rates of Alzheimer's disease are climbing, and not just because of better diagnosis. Alzheimer's shares deep metabolic roots with the top three diet-related chronic illnesses: diabetes, heart disease, and obesity.

We followed the experts' advice and cut the fat out, thinking we'd get leaner and healthier. But when we replaced the good foods with bad ones, we took a turn for the worse. So, how can we get—and stay—healthy? After years of working with two popular diets, and closely observing what worked—and more importantly, what didn't—we've found the answer.

The optimal eating plan, we've both concluded, features high levels of beneficial fat and fiber *and* the right amount of clean protein for weight loss—all bound together with delicious, healthful flavor and ample nutrients. That's the Smart Fat Solution. And here's what it looks like.

Fat

The type of fat we're advocating—smart fat—has two amazing properties, both of which contribute to effective weight loss and long-term good health.

First, smart fat *alters your hormonal balance* so that you feel more energetic and less hungry while you burn more calories. And second, smart fat *lowers your levels of inflammation,* which benefits nearly every aspect of your health.

In later chapters, we'll explain these two concepts in greater detail, but for now, we want you to know that when you seek out smart fats and combine them with fiber, protein, and flavor, you'll have a powerful weight-management tool that you can use for life. As a result, you'll feel healthy and energetic. What you *won't* feel is deprived.

Protein

The ideal diet has to have just the right amount of protein. This is particularly true when you're trying to lose weight, because protein helps you feel full and helps the body burn calories more efficiently. Before we tell you about quantity, that is, how much protein you should consume, we first want to emphasize the *quality* of protein.

When it comes to protein, quality almost always trumps quantity. You will not lose weight (and be truly healthy) unless you choose *clean*

SMART MOVE: QUICK-START YOUR SMART FAT SOLUTION

Here's a small step to help you shift your mindset as you begin this book. For now, simply remember the key ingredients in the Smart Fat Solution when you prepare a meal or want a snack: *fat, protein, fiber, and flavor*. You don't need to be rigid about combining all four ingredients every time you eat, but aim to get fat, protein, fiber, and flavor into your diet every day.

Let's say you're putting your lunch together. Pick a ripe avocado (smart fat); pair it with some organic, cage-free chicken (a clean protein); add some chickpeas, tomatoes, and cucumbers (fiber); and accent all with a dash of olive oil vinaigrette, smart fat *and* flavor. There's your meal!

Maybe you don't have a ripe avocado, or you don't particularly want one. Wild-caught salmon (clean protein) instead of chicken pairs nicely with the chickpea salad, and because the salmon contains omega-3 fatty acids—one of the "smartest" fats you can consume—you'd be combining in one food a smart fat and a clean protein. Or, how about some grass-fed beef—which in addition to being a clean protein also contains omega-3s—combined with flavorful white beans and fresh sage and garlic?

Looking for a healthy snack? Try some almonds and a bit of dark chocolate for a nutrient-packed handful of flavor, fiber, and smart fat.

As you work through this book, you'll begin to learn more about how to put together meals and snacks with these principles—fat, protein, fiber, and flavor—in mind. You'll also learn to swap out ingredients to achieve a balance and flavor profile that most appeal to you. It's easy—and best of all, it's delicious. Once you start, you'll want to smart-fat all your food—for life!

protein—we're talking organic plant protein, such as soy, beans, and protein powders; or animal protein that is organic, wild-caught, grass-fed, free-range, or pasture-raised, all of which are low in inflammatory omega-6 fatty acids. Such sources of clean protein are great for you, unlike sources of "mean" protein, which in the case of animals means grain-fed and factory-farmed. Mean protein leads to inflammation, which makes us sick and fat—the opposite of what clean protein can do for us. Remember this shorthand: Always choose protein that's *clean, not mean.* (And after we explain why, we'll teach you how to do this.)

Fiber

Fiber makes you feel full and satisfied, which sets you up for successful weight loss. Eat fiber to shed pounds, lower your blood sugar levels and blood pressure, and improve your cholesterol profile. When you combine fiber with smart fat and protein, you'll reach your weight-loss goals and lower your risk for developing many diseases.

Flavor

Believe it or not, weight loss and good food are not mutually exclusive. In fact, they're complementary. You're more likely to stick with a way of eating if you love the way your food tastes. That's right, appealing flavors are the key to weight-loss success, and—even better—excellent flavor *also* means great nutrition.

Herbs, spices, and condiments are like a natural medicine cabinet full of phytochemicals (living plant compounds) loaded with anti-aging and anti-inflammatory properties. A major part of creating flavor is how we prepare food. Marinating and grilling and other simple cooking techniques (as we'll explain later) not only enhance the flavor of your meals, but protect their nutritional value.

Putting It All Together: How to Use This Book

The Smart Fat Solution will challenge your long-held attitudes about dietary fat. In fact, it may just change your attitude about diet and food in general. We'll give you guidance on what and how to eat—with lists of fat, fiber, and protein foods; meal plans; recipes; and more—but before you get to the specifics, we want you to understand why you should eat the smart fat way.

In the next chapter, we share a lot more about smart fats—why they're the key to weight loss and good health; where to find them; and why adding fiber, clean protein, and flavor to your diet is a must. We also tell you how to start incorporating smart fats into your daily diet. Over the course of this book, you'll learn what foods to eat and which ones to stay away from—and why. You'll also learn how to make sense of the sometimes confusing nutritional information about fat, carbs, and protein.

After we give you a foundation for how and why smart fats work, we get down to details with our fat-fiber-protein guidelines; lists of foods and ingredients; a two-phase, thirty-day eating plan; and more than fifty go-to recipes. Along the way, you'll get advice on serving sizes, tips on shopping and cooking, and loads of practical information to keep you on the smart fat track, during and after the Thirty-Day Plan. Best of all, you'll see how simple it is to smart-fat all your food (without a recipe): breakfast, lunch, and dinner; your restaurant selections; your family's dinner; your traditional holiday meal; your lunch box; and much more.

You won't have to count calories, grams, and percentages, though we provide those numbers for people who want to know them. (And your family and friends *will* want to know—you're going to look and feel better than ever, so they're going to wonder what you're doing differently!) Once you've got a handle on how to smart-fat your food for life, you won't even need recipes because it will all become second nature. Finally, we go beyond diet and help you make lifestyle adjustments—exercise, stress management, better sleep—that go hand in hand with lasting weight loss and excellent health.

CHAPTER 2

Why the Smart Fat Solution Will Make You Lean and Healthy

F AT, FIBER, AND PROTEIN, served up with flavor—together, they're a powerful, natural prescription for weight loss and wellness. Now let's take a good look at each of these aspects of the Smart Fat Solution so you can better understand the role they play in controlling your weight, staying lean and trim, improving your health—and saving your life.

Smart Fats at Work

Fat can make you thin, and controlling your weight will keep you healthy. Behind this simple truth are some complex (biochemical) realities, but don't worry—we're here to make them understandable.

If you don't need to shed excess weight, congrats; you'll still reap many benefits from the Smart Fat Solution, including a reduction in the risk of various illnesses. The Smart Fat Solution will help you turn back the clock on aging. Whatever your goals, there are two big physiological reasons why adding smart fat to your diet will yield the results you want:

1. *Smart fats decrease inflammation.* Inflammation is the basis for virtually every degenerative disease *and* is a huge roadblock when it comes to permanent weight loss.
2. *Smart fats balance your hormones.* If your hormones are out of whack, it's next to impossible to lose weight or to be truly healthy.

How Smart Fats Break the Inflammation Chain

Consuming beneficial dietary fat sets off a positive biochemical reaction in our bodies, which decreases disease-causing, obesity-promoting inflammation. Don't underestimate the damage that chronic inflammation can cause.

When most of us think of "inflammation" (Latin *inflammato;* literally, "I ignite"), we picture an angry-looking rash or the swelling around a joint. Got an abscess in your tooth? An eruption on your skin? An aching back? It's inflammation—at least the kind most of us are familiar with.

Inflammation is the body's response to injury (the throbbing of your sprained ankle that blew up like a balloon) or to infection (the puffy, itching skin around your scraped knee). Your body correctly perceives that it's under attack, and in an attempt to control the damage, the immune system mounts a counterattack. If you get a splinter, the body sends fluid to the affected area, surrounding it with white blood cells to prevent microbes from invading and starting an infection. The neighboring vascular tissue goes into overdrive, trying to protect the body by kicking out the enemy—everything from bacteria to damaged cells.

This particular variety of inflammation is called *acute* inflammation. We're all familiar with acute inflammation because it's annoyingly painful and impossible to ignore. But the kind of inflammation we're talking about here is very different. The potentially lethal kind of inflammation that causes or promotes every degenerative disease known to humans is a completely different animal. This much more dangerous kind of inflammation is called *chronic* inflammation, and though it does incalculable damage to our bodies over the course of our lives, it exists largely below our pain threshold.

Like high blood pressure and diabetes, chronic inflammation has no visible symptoms (though it can be measured by a lab test known as high-sensitivity C-reactive protein [hs CRP]). But it damages the vascular system, the organs, the brain, and body tissues. It slowly erodes your health, gradually overwhelming the body's anti-inflammatory defenses. It causes heart disease. It causes cognitive decline and memory loss. Even obesity and diabetes are linked to inflammation because fat cells are veritable factories for inflammatory chemicals. In fact, it's likely that inflammation is the key link between obesity and all the diseases obesity puts you at risk for developing.

When your joints are chronically inflamed, degenerative diseases like arthritis are right around the corner. Inflamed lungs cause asthma and other respiratory illnesses. Inflammation in the brain is linked to Alzheimer's disease and other neurological conditions, including brain fog and everyday memory lapses that we write off as normal aging—except those memory lapses are *not* an inevitable consequence of aging at all. They are, however, an inevitable consequence of inflammation, because inflammation sets your brain on fire. Those "I forgot where I parked the car" moments start happening more frequently, and occurring prematurely.

Inflamed arteries can signal the onset of heart disease. Chronic inflammation has also been linked to various forms of cancer; it triggers harmful changes on a molecular level that result in the growth of cancer cells. Inflammation is so central to the process of aging and breakdown at the cellular level that some health pundits have begun referring to the phenomena as "inflam-aging." That's because inflammation *accelerates* aging, including the visible signs of aging we all see in the skin.

In addition to making us sick, chronic inflammation can make permanent weight loss fiendishly difficult. The fat cells keep churning out inflammatory proteins called *cytokines,* promoting even more inflammation. That inflammation in turn prevents the energy-making structures in the cells, called *mitochondria,* from doing their jobs efficiently, much like a heat wave would affect the output of a factory that lacks air-conditioning—productivity declines under extreme conditions. One of the duties of the mitochondria is burning fat; inflammation interferes with the job of the mitochondria, making fat burning more difficult and fat loss nearly impossible.

While someone trying to lose weight may initially be successful, after a while, the number on the scale gets stuck. The much-discussed weight-loss "plateau" is often a result of this cycle of inflammation and fat storage. And here's even more bad news: Adding more exercise or eating fewer calories in an attempt to break through the plateau will have *some* effect on weight loss, but not much. And continuing to lose weight becomes much harder to accomplish. Why? Because inflammation decreases our normal ability to burn calories. (We'll tell you more about other factors that contribute to the plateau—and how the Smart Fat Solution can help you to move beyond them—in Part 2 of this book.)

Remember, *some* inflammation is a good thing; it's part of the body's natural healing response, and it helps us recover from illness and injury. But when inflammation goes unchecked, which is the definition of chronic inflammation, watch out!

So how do we stop inflammation from harming our health and making permanent weight-loss impossible? Simple. *By fortifying our body's anti-inflammatory army.* And this begins with the consumption of anti-inflammatory foods, in particular, smart fats.

Smart Fats Fight Back

We know that certain fats have anti-inflammatory properties capable of breaking the frustrating cycle of inflammation. These smart fats include powerful anti-inflammatories like omega-3 fatty acids, which are primarily found in fish and fish oil, as well as in olive oil, nuts, dark chocolate, and avocados.

Reducing inflammation, however, is not as simple as just loading up on omega-3s, though it's definitely a first step. It's also a matter of consuming *less* inflammatory food. This is logical, but it's not always simple to do. That's because some of the "heart-healthy" fats we've been taught to consume are the worst offenders, most notably poly-unsaturated "vegetable" oils that the Diet Dictators have been touting since the birth of the low-fat diet.

These polyunsaturated fats are also known as omega-6 fatty acids. They're very common in junk foods (almost all of which are made with various forms of so-called vegetable oils), but they're also in some "healthy" foods as well. No matter where they come from, though, *omega-6 fats are pro-inflammatory.* Consuming too much omega-6,

---

SMART FAT FACT:
THERE ARE NO VEGGIES IN "VEGETABLE" OIL

Vegetable oils don't come from vegetables, so the name is misleading. They are processed from grains such as corn or from other plants such as soybeans. To distinguish these fats from animal fats, manufacturers have long referred to them as "vegetable" oil, and that's how most consumers refer to them as well. But the name is flat-out wrong. More accurately, they are plant-based oils derived from grains and seeds. We use "vegetable oil" in this book because it is common usage, but we want to point out—and we want you to understand—the inaccuracy of that term.

then, is problematic. (Note: Omega-6 is not in and of itself "bad," and we do need *some* of this essential fatty acid in our diets. The problem is that we're consuming *too much* omega-6, while consuming *too little* omega-3.)

Here's the solution: For omega-3s to counteract inflammation most effectively, they must be eaten in the correct ratio to omega-6s—ideally, about 1:1.

But that's *not* what we're doing. Research indicates that our current consumption of omega-6 fats is about sixteen times greater than our consumption of omega-3s, or roughly a ratio of 16:1. That means we're giving 1,600 percent more "fuel" to our body's *inflammatory* army than to its *anti-inflammatory* army.

As you'll see, getting this ratio right is vital. Our health depends on it—as do our very lives. While the ratio of 1:1 is the ideal, we believe that you can do just fine with a ratio of anywhere between 1:1 and 4:1. But 16:1? Not so much!

Once your ratio is calibrated, smart fats can go to work in your body and bust the cycle of inflammation to help you lose weight, fight disease, and stop accelerated aging.

THE THREE CATEGORIES OF FAT: THE GOOD, THE BAD, AND THE NEUTRAL

You can't survive without fat. It's that simple. In order to survive, your body *must have fat*.

By now, you probably understand that not all fats are created equal. Different fats work differently in our bodies. So don't run out and start ordering hamburgers and fries chased with a creamy milkshake. Just because you need to eat fat doesn't mean you get to eat fat indiscriminately. You still have to be smart about fats.

First, a quick Chemistry 101 lesson and some terminology you should know. Scientists place fats into categories on the basis of their chemical architecture, specifically, the presence of what chemists call *double bonds*. Fats that have *no* double bonds are called "saturated" fats; fats that have *one* double bond are called "*mono*unsaturated" fats; and fats that have *more than one* double bond are "*poly*unsaturated" fats. Polyunsaturated fats are further divided into omega-6s and omega-3s, named solely for the location of their first double bond.

The best (smartest) fats are those that yield clear health benefits, including weight loss. Some fats are pure junk, and the worst of them are deadly. Some fats will add flavor and texture to your daily diet, but they won't have much effect on your health. We consider those fats "neutral," and they pretty much get a free pass. Unlike smart fats, you don't need to make a special effort to add them to your diet, but you don't need to make a special effort to avoid them either.

Throughout this book, you'll hear us refer to fats as good (smart), bad (dumb), or neutral. Here are a few examples of each.

GOOD (SMART) FATS

- Olives, olive oil, avocados, most nuts (almonds, pecans, walnuts, pistachios, hazelnuts, and macadamia nuts), and seeds (chia, flax, and pumpkin)
- Fatty fish and fish oils
- Dark chocolate
- Coconut, coconut oil, and medium-chain triglyceride (MCT) oil[†]

BAD (DUMB) FATS

- Trans fats found in fast foods and packaged foods. Also called *hydrogenated* or *partially hydrogenated* oils, trans fats are biochemically similar to liquid plastic, essentially acting like embalming fluid in your tissues. Trans fats might lengthen a food's shelf life, but they will shorten *your* shelf life.

CONTINUED ON NEXT PAGE

[†] MCT oil is commercially available and usually derived from coconut and palm kernel oils. See our discussion of coconut oil in Chapter 5.

CONTINUED FROM PAGE 23

- "Vegetable" oils that have been highly refined and chemically altered through industrial processes; they're damaged fats, processed with high heat and extracted with nasty chemicals.
- Fats from animals shot full of chemicals, hormones, and pesticides. Think of these animals as toxic; their fat is equally so.
- Fats high in omega-6s, especially if they are used in foods that don't have any other redeeming benefit.

NEUTRAL FATS

- Certain (*clean*) saturated fats—such as palm oil or the fat found naturally in grass-fed and organically raised animal protein, such as beef, lard, butter, yogurt, milk, cream, and cheese. We consider these clean sources of saturated fats to be neutral. In general, neutral fats may not necessarily improve health, but they certainly won't cause any harm. We've demonized saturated fats for decades, but it turns out that they have nothing to do with what's killing us. In fact, you're much better off eating a steak from a grass-fed, organically raised animal than you are eating white rice, white potatoes, or bread. (We'll tell you what's *really* doing the damage in the next chapter.)

We've placed fats into these three categories because of how they behave biochemically once they've been ingested and go to work in our bodies. We tell you more about that in Chapter 4 when we look at fats more closely, and we also give you lots more examples of foods in all three categories.

In looking at our three distinctions, do you notice anything interesting? We're betting that foods you would most like to eat are made with fats that fall into the good and neutral categories. If you think about smart fat eating with that in mind, planning great meals and choosing satisfying snacks gets easier and easier.

How Smart Fats Keep Your Hormones in Balance

Freud wrote, "Biology is destiny." He was, of course, writing about women, but we'd like to rephrase this adage so it applies to both genders and better reflects what we now know about how our bodies work.

We would say, *biochemistry* is destiny.

Our hormones control everything—inside and out, from our appearance to our behavior. They determine how many calories we burn while working at our desk, and our cravings and appetite when we sit down to eat a meal. This is true at every age, for both genders. As we go through our natural lives, some hormones are more active than others, to be sure, but the constant biochemical reactions that hormones set off in our bodies are inevitable.

So what happens when something throws off our hormonal balancing act?

When hormones are off-kilter, all sorts of health problems ensue, ranging from mild to deadly serious. Our focus in this book is on how specific hormones affect weight gain, weight loss, and overall health—*and* why smart fats are the key to keeping your hormones balanced. Dozens of hormones circulate throughout the body, but three in particular react to smart—and dumb—fats. Though each originates from a different source, these three hormones—insulin, leptin, and cortisol—share a close relationship.

Insulin: The Traffic Cop Hormone

When it comes to weight, the hormone that gets all the glory—or the blame, depending on how you look at it—is insulin. Insulin has two nicknames, both of which tell you something about its intimate connection with your waistline: One is the "hunger hormone," and the other is the "fat-storage hormone."

As you probably know, after you eat *anything,* whether it's cauliflower or candy, your blood sugar naturally rises. In response, your pancreas secretes insulin, which acts as a kind of traffic cop for sugar, directing insulin into cells, where it's either used as energy or eventually stored as fat.

That's the abridged version; lots of other factors are at work here, and some other hormones, too. The *type* of food you eat is a big factor. Some foods have only a minor effect on blood sugar levels, while others send those levels through the roof. (And remember, the more your blood sugar goes up, the more insulin the pancreas has to secrete to manage it. The more insulin you secrete, the more likely it is you'll store fat and the less likely it is you'll burn it—and the more likely you'll suffer from accelerated aging and diseases like diabetes.)

Carbohydrates, proteins, and fats influence blood sugar in different ways. They also have different effects on the amount of insulin your pancreas releases, the rate at which insulin is released, and the fate of excess blood sugar (glucose)[†]—will it be stored as fat, or will it be burned for fuel?

Refined carbohydrates that rapidly break down into sugar have the most profound effect on insulin, stimulating the highest amount of fat storage. Protein has far less of an effect, resulting in minimal fat storage. Fat itself? Absolutely no effect.

This last point is important. Fat has *no substantial effect* on blood sugar levels, insulin secretion, or the conversion of sugar to body fat or fuel. Think about this for a minute. The class of food we've been advised to eat in high quantities (carbs) for the past four decades has a profound (and negative!) effect on insulin, the very hormone that makes us fat. But the foods we've been told to *avoid* (fats) have virtually *no* effect. The low-fat, high-refined-carb diets we've been encouraged to follow for decades are actually contributing to poor health and weight gain *because* of the havoc they wreak on insulin levels. And when insulin is chronically elevated—which is what happens when we keep driving our

---

[†] In this context, we are using the terms *blood sugar* and *glucose* interchangeably, as in "blood sugar levels" and "blood glucose levels"; *glucose* refers to the amount of sugar that can be measured in the bloodstream—sugar that our bodies produce after we consume food.

blood glucose levels up with the wrong foods—the cells stop "listening" to it, which leads to a condition known as *insulin resistance.*

Insulin resistance is almost always found in cases of obesity and type 2 diabetes. (Type 2 diabetes was once known as "adult-onset" diabetes. Not anymore. We're seeing it now in twelve-year-olds!) Under normal circumstances, insulin tells your muscle cells to store energy as glycogen, the storage form of glucose. That glycogen serves as fuel for the muscles to use during their next workout, just as your car's gas tank holds the fuel for your next car ride.

But when you're insulin-resistant, those signals don't get through. And the first cells to stop responding to insulin are the muscle cells. This is especially true if you're sedentary: Your diet keeps spiking your blood sugar and insulin levels, but your muscle cells need less and less glycogen because you're sitting around at a desk all day! And because your body won't burn off this fat, you're going to get fatter and fatter.

But the bad news doesn't end there, because insulin resistance doesn't just affect our body and our fat stores. It has a major impact on our brains as well.

You see, insulin is also vital for normal brain function. Your brain needs glucose—or some form of energy—just like your muscles do. But when brain cells stop "listening" to insulin, insulin's knock at the brain cells' doors goes unanswered. Your blood sugar rises, insulin tries to deliver the sugar for energy, yet the cells aren't opening their doors and the sugar can't get in. This is insulin resistance in the brain. Cognitive performance begins to suffer. So does memory. If your blood sugar remains high, your brain is eventually damaged and even begins to atrophy. This is why researchers like Suzanne de La Monte refer to Alzheimer's disease as "type 3 diabetes."

Insulin resistance—triggered by consuming too many dietary carbohydrates—causes your body to store too much fat while at the same time interfering with your brain's ability to utilize glucose. Sugary and starchy carbs such as corn, potatoes, and rice send insulin levels up so high that the cells stop hearing its message. It's like getting used to loud ambient noise—after a while you just don't notice it. (We talk more about insulin resistance and the condition known as Metabolic Syndrome in Chapter 4.) The point is that insulin greatly affects weight control, brain health, *and* overall wellness—and eating the wrong food sends your insulin levels in the wrong direction.

If you want to keep your insulin levels in balance—and thereby reduce the risk of obesity, diabetes, heart disease, cancer, Alzheimer's, and more—eat more of the one macronutrient that won't have a negative effect on this important hormone: *fat.*

Neutral fats don't affect insulin activity one way or the other. Dumb fats make insulin resistance worse. But smart fats *reduce* insulin resistance. They help make your tissues more insulin-*sensitive*—which is exactly what you want them to be.

Leptin: The Fuel Meter Hormone

Leptin is like the gas gauge in your car. When you're driving on "low" and heading toward "empty," your gauge warns that it's time to fill 'er up. When you've got enough in the tank, you can drive normally until your gauge indicates it's time to pull over and get more fuel. But if the gas gauge is broken, you're in trouble.

In your body, leptin works in a similar manner—at least when it's functioning as it should. It lets your brain know how much you've got left in your tank (how much energy you have stored in your fat cells) and when you need to make a pit stop (eat some food!). Leptin is released by the fat cells in proportion to how full they are, and when the hormone is working properly, it allows you to naturally monitor your food intake. When leptin is high, it's like an "off" switch on your appetite: It tells your brain that you're full and should stop eating. When leptin is low, the opposite happens: The brain gets the signal that you're hungry, and you crave food.

It's quite an elegant system. That is, when it's working. When it's not, it's like driving with a busted gas gauge.

When your gas gauge doesn't work, you have no idea when you're about to run out of fuel. You might be hovering right around "empty," but then again, you might not be. If you're smart, you pull over and pump in more gas, "just in case." (Who wouldn't?)

Now imagine what would happen if your leptin "gauge" malfunctioned. You wouldn't know when to eat *or* when to put the fork down. You'd probably want to do the eating equivalent of "fill 'er up" at every pit stop, "just in case." If your leptin function is "broken," you will overeat (just in case). Your brain is no longer getting the message that you're full, and in fact, you may well feel hungry all the time. You won't know when to stop. You'll gain weight.

(Note: If you choose to crash diet, you also mess with your leptin function. When you undereat on purpose, you're telling your metabolism to "slow down," meaning that your body will now learn how to effectively run on fewer calories. When you eventually *do* return to "normal" eating—because you can't crash diet forever—your fat cells will hang on to what they now see as "surplus" calories and you'll start packing on body fat, regaining all the weight you thought you lost for good.)

So leptin levels are sky high, but the cells are deaf to the hormone's message. It's as if leptin were trapped behind a soundproof glass door, screaming at the brain, *"You're full, you're full!"* but the brain can't hear a thing. And if that image seems familiar, it's because that's almost exactly what happens with insulin resistance. You'll recall that with insulin resistance the cells stop "listening" to insulin. When the cells stop "listening" to leptin, it's called *leptin resistance.* Insulin resistance and leptin resistance tend to travel together; if you've got one, chances are you've got both.

And that's a big problem.

Both insulin resistance and leptin resistance can be triggered by eating excessive amounts of refined carbohydrates. Junky carbs—through a long chain of events—wind up making you store increasing amounts of fat in your fat cells. Those plumped-up fat cells will then release more leptin in an attempt to send your brain a message that might sound something like this:

Dear Brain:
Just another reminder that we've had enough food for now,
thanks. We know you like donut holes, but we don't need any.
Like we keep saying, we're stuffed. Didn't Leptin deliver our last
message? Have you heard from him? Is he falling down on the
job? We'll send him out again, just in case.
   — Your Friends, the Fat Cells

Remember, when the system is working as it should, balanced levels of leptin will tell you to quit eating because you're full. But once again, as with insulin resistance, when the system isn't working, the hormonal message isn't getting through. In this case, it's the brain that isn't receiving the signal because its leptin receptors are overwhelmed:

Hey, Brain:
HELLO! We keep sending up Leptin to tell you to shut your trap,
you've had enough to eat, but clearly you aren't getting our
messages. For goodness sake, will you quit sending us those
donut holes? We keep telling you we don't want them, and we
certainly don't need them . . . but as long as they're here, mmmm,
we'll take another half dozen . . . but seriously, no more after
this! Brain, please let us know whether you're getting any of our
messages! It looks like they're going to your spam folder! We'll
try sending Leptin again. Our jeans are getting tighter by the
minute!
   — Impatiently yours (and growing daily), the Fat Cells

So, how do you keep your leptin gauge in good working order? By fueling your tank with the right stuff—smart fat. Smart fats and clean protein—especially when combined with a high-fiber and low-sugar/low-starch diet—will cause your leptin levels to rise naturally (think of that needle on the gas gauge after you fuel up). You'll feel satisfied, *and* you'll stop eating when you should. If you are eating bad fat, especially combined with sugary and starchy carbs (think donut holes), you're literally sugaring your gas tank and disrupting the whole leptin messaging system. Smart fats will set things right, and your brain will never miss an important message again.

Cortisol: The Fight-or-Flight Hormone

Cortisol is the major stress hormone in the body. Like adrenaline, it's produced by the adrenal glands in response to stress, whether that stress comes from being chased by a grizzly bear or being stuck in traffic (and being late to work, where the boss is waiting). Like insulin and leptin, the release of cortisol sets off a chain reaction that can harm both brain and body if cortisol levels become too high for sustained periods of time and therefore unmanageable.

Let's go back to that grizzly (or the traffic jam and the clock-watching boss, who is a twenty-first-century grizzly—your body doesn't know the difference). In both cases you're stressed. Your adrenal glands release some cortisol—also known as the "fight or flight" hormone, because it helps prepare your body for a defensive action, such as picking up a club to fight off the bear or running like crazy for the nearest tree. That's why cortisol, in the proper amounts, is *absolutely necessary* for survival.

The first thing cortisol does is make your blood sugar level rise; after all, you're going to need energy, and right now, that's your body's main concern. Cortisol doesn't particularly care where that sugar is coming from; it just needs to make sure there's plenty of it. Cortisol also couldn't care less what happens to all the leftover sugar still hanging out in your bloodstream after you've safely fled from the bear (or the boss's office). Like the firefighter spraying a zillion gallons of water on a dangerous fire, cortisol just wants to get the job done—in this case, making sure plenty of sugar is available for your cells so you can survive this emergency.

If you eat a lot of nutrient-poor carbohydrates—such as white bread, white rice, and sugar—and bad fats, and at the same time you *don't* eat enough clean protein, smart fat, and healthy fiber, your cortisol machinery gets all screwed up. Any form of stress—be it a bear, the boss, a family argument, or a deficient diet—triggers a release of cortisol. And ultimately, that leads to higher blood sugar levels *and* excess glucose, which, as you know, will inevitably be converted to fat.

Even worse, if your stress levels are high because of day-to-day lifestyle factors that you can't easily avoid or control (such as a precarious work situation or a difficult relationship), your adrenal glands are primed to work overtime. Imagine that your cortisol levels are already elevated because you're facing something stressful, such as caring for a sick parent while trying to balance the demands of your work and personal lives. Your cortisol remains high just because of your 24/7 caregiving role. Unfortunately, the more stress you have, the more cortisol you'll produce, and the more cortisol you produce, the greater the threat to your weight and health.

In addition to causing an imbalance in blood sugar, high cortisol levels have been linked to

- Increased abdominal fat (a marker for Metabolic Syndrome, or prediabetes)
- Decreased bone density and muscle mass
- Poor immune function
- Increased appetite and cravings
- Increased depression and anxiety
- Lower cognitive function (the memory center of your brain will literally shrink)
- Increased growth of arterial plaque and risk for heart disease

Plus, let's be realistic. After an awful, stressful day, do you feel like eating "something healthy," let alone cooking it? No. (There's a reason that ice cream, cookies, alcohol, and potato chips are called "comfort foods"!) So not only is stress harmful to your physiology, it *also* makes it difficult for you to make good decisions. This is why it's virtually impossible to lose weight and attain good health without first learning how to deal with stress. Stress is *not* all in your head. It powerfully affects your hormones, which in turn negatively affects your waistline, your brain, and your overall health. That's why we devote Chapter 9 to managing stress and other related lifestyle factors that can influence hormonal balance.

For now, let's just say that a good diet can do wonders to normalize your three primary hormones. When you eat a diet rich in smart fats, clean protein, and fiber—while avoiding lots of nutrient-poor, factory-made carbs and dumb fats—you'll be prepared to deal with all those stressors, big and small, that kick-start abnormal cortisol production.

GOOD FAT AND GOOD SEX: ARE YOU GETTING ENOUGH?

We've told you about three hormones—insulin, leptin, and cortisol—that have a major effect on weight control and general health, and why a diet rich in smart fat helps regulate blood sugar and keep things in balance. But three other important hormones also have big roles in determining your weight and your well-being: testosterone, estrogen, and progesterone, collectively known as the *sex hormones*.

Testosterone, the male sex hormone, is produced naturally from cholesterol, as are the female hormones progesterone and estrogen. When we lower our cholesterol levels by excessively reducing smart fat (or when prescribed cholesterol-reducing statin drugs), a seldom discussed side effect is that we often inadvertently lower our testosterone—and our libidos, too. Unfortunately, the body can make only so much testosterone. Just eating more cholesterol won't raise your testosterone; if only it were that easy, but it's not. And if we dramatically lower our cholesterol, since we're no longer producing enough of our crucial sex hormones, we're probably also decreasing our fertility rates.

Statin drugs have been shown to lower testosterone in men by fifty

CONTINUED ON NEXT PAGE

CONTINUED FROM PAGE 33

to seventy points. Sure, you can take a pill for erectile dysfunction, and if you're trying to start a family (whether you're male or female), modern medicine is standing by with a range of fertility treatments. But in many cases, it may just be a matter of making sure you aren't depriving yourself of adequate smart fats.

It works the other way, too. If you consume a diet of dumb fats—like trans fats and fats from animal products full of hormones and pesticides—you're harming your sexual and reproductive health. Obesity is linked to hormone dysfunction and low fertility in both men and women. It also means that you are carrying around extra weight that is probably making you extra self-conscious—never a good thing when it comes to sexual intimacy. Plus, it makes you extra averse to exercising for fitness and general well-being.

And whether it's because of too much dumb fat or too little smart fat, the same mechanism has been triggered: Your diet is throwing your sex hormones out of whack. You may be feeling inactive in and out of the bedroom, but your fat cells aren't—they're busy converting testosterone to estrogen, in women *and* in men.

For men, this means lower testosterone. For women, this means excessive estrogen in relation to progesterone, a surefire way to disrupt many stages of reproductive health, from fertility through menopause, with irregular periods, weight gain, mood swings, and serious health consequences. The risk of uterine cancer, for instance, has been linked to high levels of estrogen in relation to progesterone, a condition known, not surprisingly, as *estrogen dominance*.

Whether you're male or female, younger or older, keep in mind that what you eat at any phase in your life affects the balance of sex hormones in your body. A healthy and satisfying sex life starts with a healthy and satisfying diet—which means a diet rich in smart fats.

Fiber Power

If you were going to make only one change to your diet, we'd probably recommend this: *Eat more fiber.* Fiber is awesome, and very much underappreciated (probably because of its unglamorous association with "making you regular"). Its many benefits include the following:

- It suppresses appetite and cravings and helps you feel full (so you eat less).
- It dampens the rise in your blood sugar and insulin levels after a meal.
- It decreases inflammation.
- It lowers blood pressure.
- It improves your cholesterol profile.
- It helps remove toxins from your system.
- It feeds the healthy bacteria in your gut (the microbiome).

Fiber is also an excellent way to reduce the risks of developing heart disease and diabetes, and it can turn back the clock on aging. Plus, dietary fiber is a powerful ally in weight loss, *particularly* when it's part of a smart fat diet. Oh yes, and it really *does* keep you regular.

Why Fiber Should Be a Part of Your Daily Diet

We think that just about all forms of fiber from nutrient-dense sources— like whole, fresh produce; nuts and seeds; beans and legumes; a few types of starches; and fiber supplements, like ground flaxseed and chia seeds—are good for you. Scientists label fiber as either *soluble* (meaning it dissolves in water) or *insoluble.* We aren't particularly concerned with those labels right now, which apply more to how fiber behaves in a laboratory setting. What matters to us is how fiber performs *in your body,* particularly as part of the Smart Fat Solution. Soluble or insoluble, fiber belongs on your plate today, for the following reasons.

Fiber Helps You Lose Weight

Fiber fills you up—literally. If you eat a bowl of steel-cut oatmeal with a shot of protein powder and topped with berries and almonds for breakfast, you aren't going to be hungry when you head into that late-morning meeting. Instead, you'll be satisfied, with plenty of fuel in your tank to spare. (If you've never mixed protein powder into your oats, it's as easy as it sounds—see "Pick Your Powder: Whey to Go!" in Chapter 5 for more information.) Likewise, if you top your salad with some chickpeas at lunch, thanks to the extra fiber and protein, we can guarantee that you won't feel hungry an hour later. Have a heaping portion of roasted asparagus at dinner and you'll round out your meal, not your backside.

Fiber-rich solid foods take longer to chew, which allows your body to get the signal to your brain that your hunger is being dealt with—no need to overeat. And, because of their bulk, fiber-rich foods also take longer to digest and absorb than flimsier food choices, leaving you satisfied for much longer. An apple and a handful of nuts will satiate your hunger; a big bag of chips won't, even though the chips have more calories (and far fewer nutrients). And with high-fiber foods, you'll have fewer cravings, more energy, *and* you'll be less likely to overeat at your next meal, or worse, make a bad snack choice to tide you over until the next meal.

Fiber Makes You "Regular" in More Ways Than One

As we've seen, spikes in blood sugar send your hormones running for cover or straight into battle, but high-fiber foods actually help lower and normalize your blood sugar, which allows your hormones to stabilize and function normally. This is critical. You already know what happens when blood sugar goes up too fast and stays high too long. All that extra sugar in your bloodstream goes lookin' for love in all the wrong places, like your fat cells (like your love handles). But when you eat high-fiber foods, that doesn't happen. That's because the dietary fiber in a serving of blueberries or a bowl of steel-cut oats acts

FOOD (CARBS) FOR THOUGHT

All fiber-rich foods are classified as carbohydrates, but not all carbohydrates are rich in fiber. Far from it. Though sometimes found together, carbs and fiber are quite different animals—they are not all created equal—and their effect on your body is very different.

Certain carbs—like so-called healthy whole-grain breads, crackers, and breakfast cereals—do contain a little bit of fiber, but most likely less than you might think.

We think that you should ban from your diet any processed carbohydrate foods. Period. Fake health foods like that commercially manufactured "multigrain" pretzel are just not worth eating. They are filled with the very quick-release carbs that wreak havoc on your blood sugar and set off metabolic mayhem. We'll talk more about this type of carbohydrate in the chapters to come, but for now, think of it this way: If you grind a grain into flour, it acts just like sugar.

Eat more beans and legumes, nuts and seeds, low-sugar vegetables, low-sugar fruits, and a few select grains in small portions, such as steel-cut oatmeal, wild rice, and quinoa. (Technically, quinoa is a seed, but it looks, cooks, and tastes like a grain; plus it has the added advantage of being gluten-free.) All these foods are considered carbohydrates, but they're definitely "good" carbs, and they're great sources of fiber. Stay tuned for a discussion of "good" versus "bad" carbs in Chapter 4, where we also tell you why some fruits may be better picks than others. We love fresh, whole fruit, but berries, for example, are a better choice than a ripe banana, and you will know why once you understand the role of a food's *glycemic load,* rather than its *glycemic index.*

as a kind of brake. With fiber, your body releases insulin more slowly than it does when you eat junky carbs, even junky carbs that claim to contain fiber, like "whole-grain" crackers. Eat a brownie or a bagel and you may feel a burst of temporary energy, but it'll be like what they say about Chinese food—an hour later you'll be hungry. Meanwhile, you've got some extra glucose heading straight for your fat cells, which are more than happy to fling open their doors. Eat more fiber, and this doesn't happen. You'll have long-lasting energy, plus you'll feel and look much better.

Fiber Keeps You Healthy for the Long Haul

Fiber can help you *get* thin and *stay* thin. We recently authored an abstract that was presented at the American College of Nutrition meeting (in November 2015), focusing on which lifestyle changes impact weight loss. Want to know what we presented as the No. 1 best predictor of long-term weight loss? Fiber intake. Eating more fiber helps you lose weight long term. The second best predictor is adding more exercise minutes per week. So if you only want to make one change to lose weight and keep it off—eat more fiber!

It can also help you live a longer, healthier life. It lowers your blood pressure, it improves your cholesterol profile, *and* it reduces inflammation. Substances found in fiber-filled foods—such as *anthocyanins* (the bright blue/purple pigments in blueberries and cherries), *lycopene* (the red pigments in tomatoes and watermelon), *lutein* (in kale), and *beta-carotene* (in butternut squash)—are powerful antioxidant compounds that also protect your heart. These compounds decrease the stiffening of arteries that occurs with age, lower your blood pressure, and prevent arterial plaque from forming.

Fibrous foods like beans block cholesterol from being absorbed into the bloodstream—actually, beans are also the most effective food ever studied to block tissue oxidation. (Think of oxidation as a kind of internal "rusting" that contributes to inflammation and accelerated aging. Fibrous plant foods such as vegetables, fruits, beans, and nuts also contain powerful anti-inflammatories to help you fight degenerative diseases, including cancer and age-related declines in memory.)

Foods High in Fiber Do Double (and Even Triple) Duty

Nuts, seeds, and avocados are not only an excellent source of fiber, they also qualify as smart fat. Beans and legumes—our top picks for fiber—*also* provide protein. You can always find a fiber-rich food that works at breakfast, lunch, and dinner or for a snack.

Many popular weight-loss diets inadvertently steer you away from fiber-rich foods by focusing on foods higher in protein. These diets advise you to eat fewer carbohydrates, which can be a good thing if the diets cut the refined carbs and maintain the fiber; but it's not the whole story. People who follow these diets frequently wind up leaving out many nutrient-dense, fiber-rich foods, such as fresh vegetables, nuts, and beans. Most, if not all, of their calories come from protein and fat.

With the Smart Fat Solution, however, you'll eat a selection of fats, protein, *and* fiber—all without counting calories. We will never steer you away from the lifelong benefits of eating high-quality plant fiber, and we believe that following any diet that eliminates foods rich in fiber is a big mistake.

Clean Protein (for a Lean Body)

There's no magic bullet when it comes to weight loss, but protein comes pretty darn close. When you combine protein with smart fat and fiber, you're on your way to losing more weight than you've ever imagined. You're also on your way to making your body leaner, stronger, and healthier, because protein increases your metabolism and makes you a more efficient calorie-burner—even while you're sitting at your desk. Even better, protein makes you feel satisfied so you don't give in to junk food cravings. And protein helps repair nearly every cell in your body.

Though you don't need as much protein as some people think, you *do* need between 80 and 120 grams a day, depending on your age, gender, level of activity, and body composition. It's a good idea to start your day by revving up your metabolism with protein, especially if you're interested in weight loss.

Flavor, the Life Saver

Every second of every day, people fall off of their diets. The diet may be too restrictive. The food may be too difficult to find and prepare. It may be too challenging to eat well during a typical workday. The weekends are one giant pitfall of snacking and overeating. All this plays out to the soundtrack of "I'll Start Over on Monday" and is accompanied by a heaping portion of guilt—a great excuse for a mood-lifting side of onion rings.

We think the main reason that people fall off the diet wagon is this: *They don't like their food.*

Let's face it. A dinner of plain baked chicken and steamed broccoli may sound guilt-free, but it's also *flavor*-free. And who's going to look forward to eating that? Even hospital food is more appealing than what you'll find in the menu plans of some diets. And the pleasant surprise is this: That same chicken and broccoli would have had far more nutrients and been better for your health if it had had more of the right type of fantastic flavor, too. If we prepare chicken and broccoli for dinner, for instance, we make succulent roasted chicken with Mediterranean herbs and broccoli with a "smart" lemon-butter sauce. (See our recipes for both in this book!)

We love the pleasures of good food, and we think everything you eat should taste terrific. Remember: One of us—Steven—trained at the Four Seasons in Seattle to be a chef! All the foods we recommend in the Smart Fat Solution, from basic ingredients to entire meals, plus all of our recipes are designed to please your taste buds because we know that if you don't like what you're eating, you aren't going to stick with it. The best part of all this is that the very herbs and spices that happen to make food taste amazing are loaded with nutrients that will make you healthier and help you lose weight. Talk about a double whammy!

We promise to make meal planning and preparation simple. The Smart Fat Solution offers food that is delicious and easy to make. Great flavor is the key!

The Cure Is in the Spice Rack, *Not* the Medicine Cabinet

Dried or fresh, herbs and spices don't just punch up the flavor—they also boost health and fight accelerated aging. They can foil *oxidation,* a damaging chemical process in our bodies that alters and destroys our cell structure. A perfect example of oxidation, or oxidative damage, is the formation of rust when oxygen interacts with metal. The same sort of damage happens inside our bodies. In fact, the "free radical theory of aging" holds that aging is basically a kind of internal rusting. And when oxidative damage combines with inflammation, look out! That deadly combo turbo charges the aging process and causes life-threatening illness.

Enter spices and herbs. In addition to making your food scrumptious, most spices are enormously high in antioxidants and anti-inflammatories—an overlooked and underappreciated weapon in the war against chronic diseases.

To say that our global food supply has undergone major degradations in the past few centuries is an understatement. We live in a time of factory farms, pesticide use, chemical additives, genetically modified organisms (GMOs), and hydroponic greenhouses bigger than Delaware turning out thousands of tasteless tomatoes in January. Our great-grandparents wouldn't recognize many of the foods we find today in a typical supermarket, including some items in the produce aisle, such as supersweet corn.

But one constant in the way we eat hasn't changed much ever since early foodies figured out that a hunk of meat tastes way better if you *season* it before you throw it on the fire. And that's the use of spices.

Ancient civilizations were on to things like cardamom (for easing digestion), sage (an Ayurvedic "purifying" herb in traditional Indian medicine), parsley (for detoxifying and deodorizing), and cumin (for decreasing allergy symptoms—and for keeping chickens from leaving their yards). Many legendary benefits are linked to certain herbs and spices; some of them may be tall tales (like vampire-repelling garlic), but there is no doubt that even in this era of Big Food, the integrity of pure herbs and spices remains fairly unchanged. These plant foods hold tremendous value as an untapped source of disease prevention and overall well-being. Here are some of our favorite flavors, which we encourage you to use liberally to enliven your smart fat, fiber, and protein foods.

Garlic

Garlic is one of the greatest medicinal foods of all time and is definitely at the top of our list. It has a remarkable ability to lower blood pressure, prevent blood clots, and improve the blood cholesterol profile.

Allicin is the compound that gives this immune-boosting food—which has even been shown to combat symptoms of the common cold—its medicinal properties. Allicin is also responsible for garlic's fragrant aroma (the one that vampires apparently don't like). To get the most allicin from garlic, make sure you crush, press, or chop the cloves to fully release and activate this substance. Allicin is formed only when the garlic is smashed or crushed and the enzyme allinin mixes with oxygen; so in case you were so inclined, swallowing a clove of garlic whole wouldn't do you much good. When cooking, avoid overheating garlic because you not only wind up with a bitter flavor, but you also destroy its medicinal properties. Whether you like Asian, Latin, Mediterranean, or other flavors, work a clove or two of garlic

into foods such as stir-fried dishes, salad dressings, soups, and more—
and do it as often as possible.

Green Herbs

It's astounding how easy it is to get your hands on organic, fresh
green herbs throughout the entire year. They are easy to grow at home
on a south-facing windowsill even in winter, or in containers on a bal-
cony or patio if you don't "garden" on a larger scale. Growing your own
herbs is an inexpensive way to ensure a constant supply. If you can't do
this, fresh, dried varieties work beautifully.

Chewing on a sprig of **parsley** doesn't just freshen your breath; it
purifies and rejuvenates your entire system because of the high levels
of chlorophyll it contains. Studies have linked chlorophyll to everything from stopping bacterial growth to counteracting inflammation
to lowering blood sugar.

Rosemary has been linked to improved memory and brain function because it contains substances that help to protect *acetylcholine,*
a vital neurotransmitter. The prescription drug donepezil (sold under
the brand name Aricept), which is used to treat Alzheimer's disease,
works exactly the same way: by stopping the breakdown of acetylcholine. Rosemary is also a potent anti-inflammatory compound and is
often used to treat arthritis.

Sage lowers blood pressure and has an antidiabetic effect in animals. These benefits have yet to be confirmed in humans, but we do
know that sage contains anti-inflammatory substances and is an antioxidant. For centuries, it has been used in Ayurvedic medicine as a
purifying herb because of its antibacterial and antiviral properties.

Thyme, which contains an oil called *thymol,* has anti-inflammatory,
antioxidant, and antiseptic properties and aids in digestion.

Oregano also contains thymol and is considered the herb with
the highest antioxidant activity—four times higher per gram than
that of blueberries. In addition to thymol, oregano contains *carvacrol*
(another oil), which has antifungal, antibacterial, and antiparasitic

properties. Together, these anti-inflammatory substances make oregano one of the most beneficial herbs you can add to your diet.

Don't forget other herbs such as mint, chives, basil, dill, and cilantro, just to name a few. Mix and match to find the flavors that please your palate and make you healthier.

Savory Spices

Humans are biochemically drawn to certain flavors, like bees to nectar. And nature makes us attracted to these foods for good reasons. Unlike most animals, we humans can't make our own vitamin C, and many researchers theorize that our attraction to sugar is actually nature's way of getting us to eat high-in-vitamin-C foods like sweet-tasting fruits. We're also naturally primed to love most spices. Perhaps nature gave them their appealing scents so that we would eat them and enjoy all their beneficial health properties. After all, spices, by weight, are perhaps the most nutrient-dense substances we can eat. Here are a few that have been specifically linked to improved metabolism.

Cardamom, an ancient spice that you'll find in Indian cooking, is often used as a digestive aid and a breath freshener. But it also stimulates the flow of bile, which enhances liver health and fat metabolism.

Cinnamon contains phytochemicals that increase glucose metabolism in cells (and when glucose is metabolized, it doesn't get stored as fat). It also can help to lower blood sugar, decrease blood pressure, and reduce triglyceride levels and "bad" (low-density lipoprotein [LDL]) cholesterol.

Ginger helps control nausea, but it also decreases the stickiness of blood, which helps to prevent blood clots, and decreases inflammation. In animal studies, it lowered cholesterol and slowed the development of atherosclerosis.

Turmeric contains *curcumin,* one of the most powerful compounds in the plant kingdom. Curcumin has been used at the University of Texas MD Anderson Cancer Center in cancer trials. It's being studied in memory loss research at Columbia University Medical Center (it was shown to slow memory loss in laboratory animals) and at the University of California. It's extremely healthy for the liver, which is "ground zero" for detoxification. Curcumin has also been shown to improve arthritis symptoms, not surprising in view of its enormous anti-inflammatory firepower. (Both of us take curcumin in supplement form; see more on supplements in Chapter 8.)

The research on the benefits of herbs and spices continues, but there is no question that flavoring dishes with these substances can boost the health quotient of our food. Most importantly, it means that we'll stick with eating the best possible diet for life. Don't limit yourself to these flavors; we just wanted to point out those that we believe will complement the Smart Fat Solution. Experiment to your heart's content. Your body and mind will thank you.

Smart fats, clean protein, and fiber, all wrapped up in flavors that will encourage you to eat this way forever—these are the key ingredients that will make you leaner and healthier. Smart fats are the cornerstone, battling disease-causing inflammation and helping your hormones function the way they were meant to. Fiber is a nutritional powerhouse that will help you turn back the clock on aging, as it works to lower your risk of developing certain illnesses. Clean protein turns you into a formidable calorie-burner. Flavor will keep you on track because eating this way will be pleasurable. These are the lifesaving foods that we should be eating every day. Now, let's look at what we should avoid, and why.

CHAPTER 3

What *Not* to Eat

WHEN YOU FOLLOW the Smart Fat Solution, you will never run out of appealing and healthful options to eat. You don't have to be rigid about combining fat, fiber, protein, and flavor for every meal or snack, though in time, you'll naturally find yourself including all four in every meal because they taste so great together. In no time at all, you'll get the hang of putting together sensible meals and snacks without having to think twice about how to give your food a smart fat makeover. Nor will you have to worry about portion sizes or measuring grams or counting calories. The variety, and ease, of delicious foods available to you will free you once and for all from the dreaded cycle of dieting and then gaining again and having to diet again.

But before we get to the how-to (and the all-important how-*much*), let's look at the what-*not,* as in what you shouldn't put on your plate or in your mouth. Some foods on our "don't eat" list, such as artificial trans fats, won't surprise you. But we'll bet some of the others will.

Both of us have always believed that information is power. That's why we think it's important that you understand the reasons why we want you to avoid certain foods. We believe that if you understand why these changes are important—why, in fact, your life depends on making them—then you'll be much more willing to make the health changes at the heart of the Smart Fat Solution.

Fats: Not Always Okay

Despite what you may have heard, saturated fat, on its own, isn't going to kill you, though it won't necessarily improve your health. However, there's one big exception: the toxic fat found in commercially produced animal products, which, sadly, make up most of what you'll find in the meat and dairy sections of most supermarkets and in restaurants.

How Fat Moves from Being "Neutral" to Being "Bad"

The use of pesticides, hormones, and other chemicals in our food supply is rampant, and animals being raised on grains filled with these substances aren't the only ones who suffer from such an unnatural diet. All those toxic compounds are stored in the fatty tissues of the factory-farmed cow, pig, lamb, chicken, or other animal, and these toxins enter our systems when we eat such animals. And it's not just the chemicals that are a problem. It's the grain itself, too. As you'll see, a steady diet of grain, not grass, results in meat and dairy that's full of inflammatory omega-6 fats, adding to the imbalance between inflammatory omega-6s and anti-inflammatory omega-3s—an imbalance that makes us sick and keeps us from losing weight. Here are two reasons to stop eating meat and dairy products that come from grain-fed animals.

1. *Toxins in Our Food Supply (and in Our Bodies)*

Our food chain is simple and straightforward. As the saying goes, "We are what we eat." But sadly, that's not always a good thing. Take grains, for instance. Even before specific grains are fed to animals, they are treated with pesticides like Round-Up as part of the process of making feed. Compounds known as *dioxins* are chemical by-products of industrial processes. They are among the most potent carcinogens on earth, and they're in our food supply. Beef, for instance, contains the highest concentration of these deadly dioxins, but they're also found in poultry and dairy products, as well as in farmed fish.

In addition, commercial farmers add growth hormones to the feed, largely genetically modified corn and soy (all soaked through with pesticides), loaded with antibiotics in order to yield more pounds of meat for the market. Hormones also increase milk production in dairy cows. But certain growth hormones, and pesticides, have been shown to cause cancer in lab animals. These carcinogenic substances, many of which are banned in the European Union, Japan, and other developed nations, are routinely used in the United States.

Do these additives cause cancer in humans? Let's look at one example. There are no lab studies examining the relationship between rBGH, the bovine growth hormone used to increase milk production, and cancer cell growth in humans. But we do know that lab animals exposed to rBGH display elevated levels of the hormone IGF-1 (insulin-like growth factor-1). In humans, high IGF-1 is often linked to breast and colon cancers. Fortunately, there has been a public push-back against rBGH—enough to cause some U.S. milk producers to reduce, and in many cases eliminate, this hormone from their production processes. But many other potentially harmful hormones, pesticides, and chemicals that aren't as well-known as rBGH continue to find their way into our food.

Antibiotics are also part of the toxic mix. Added to the food supply of livestock, antibiotics ensure that animals stay "healthy" and gain weight faster in a crowded feedlot or chicken coop, where some level of disease is inevitable. Because of the massive numbers of animals involved in commercial operations, sick or at-risk animals are not singled out for treatment with antibiotic drugs. They are given to *all* animals. The overuse of antibiotics, in animals and in humans, results in the development of drug-resistant strains of dangerous bacteria. Imagine being seriously ill with a bacterial infection, but no effective treatment is available because the "superbug" that is making you supersick is resistant to antibiotics. This isn't a plot from a science fiction movie—it's reality.

Note that the toxic residue in fat is not limited to meat. Dairy products are similarly polluted with pesticides and chemicals. The easiest way to protect against harmful toxins is to go organic, purchasing meat and dairy products that come from pasture-raised animals.

2. *Grain-Fed Animals = Inflammatory Fats in Humans*

Grain-fed animals in industrial meat and dairy operations generally eat a diet of corn- and soy-based feed, which is packed with omega-6 fats. Grain makes for a cheap diet that fattens up confined animals quickly. But this diet is completely at odds with nature, which would have cows, pigs, sheep, and other animals grazing naturally on grass. When we consume meat, milk, eggs, butter, yogurt, cheese, and other products from grain-fed animals, we're adding inflammatory omega-6s to our plate. According to one study, grain-fed beef on average contains a ratio of omega-6s to omega-3s of 7.7:1.

Conversely, free-ranging chickens, turkeys, and other birds eat anything they come across in their yards—seeds, bugs, slugs, grass, scraps, nuts, and worms. (Yes, even some grain, but it's only a tiny part of a healthy and varied diet.) Like their four-legged barnyard neighbors, they aren't meant to be penned or caged indoors, nor raised on feed made from corn and soy. Unlike grain-fed beef, grass-fed beef has an almost perfect ratio of omega-6s to omega-3s of 1.5:1. To reduce our risk of inflammation and countless health and weight problems, choose meat and dairy products from grass-fed cows.

Certainly, organic beef is better than nonorganic because at least you won't be consuming the toxins from the pesticide-sprayed grains the cows were fed. But the unhealthy ratio of omega-6s to omega-3s is the same. Only with grass-fed meat do you get both the absence of toxins *and* a much less inflammatory fatty acid ratio.

This book is not about the ethics of the industrial production of meat and dairy products, nor the environmental impact of factory-farm operations that are spreading across the globe. (Meat consumption in China has risen dramatically as wages have increased, resulting in the creation of massive factory-farm operations for pork and chicken, with red meat becoming more popular.) It's not about the mistreatment of animals in our food chain, though we both firmly believe that much more can and should be done to improve the conditions under which animals are raised before they're taken to market.

This book is about eating smarter and eating better. So it's impossible to ignore the fact that the demand for cheap, available meat and dairy products drives the quick-and-dirty processing of grain-fed land animals, not to mention the dumbing down of smart fats. When fat slides from being neutral to being bad, we pay the price with our health (even if the prices at the supermarket or the fast-food drive-through are lower). That's the bad news, but the good news is that you do have options.

Smart Move: Eat Clean, Not Mean

If you want to avoid ingesting hormones, pesticides, and other toxins, as well as high levels of inflammatory omega-6 fats, opt for meat and dairy produced from organic pasture-raised animals. Switch from eating *mean*—dirty fats—and choose *clean*. It's that simple. Don't let these common excuses complicate this important choice.

"It's Hard to Find"

It's less and less true that healthful choices are hard to find. Unless you live in the middle of nowhere (and thanks to the Internet, no one lives *there* anymore), you probably are close to a grocery store that has a selection of grass-fed beef and other land animal protein, as well as organic, pasture-raised dairy. If your local store doesn't have any options, talk to the store manager; chances are that you aren't the only shopper in search of healthier choices. You can also research when and where the nearest farmer's market sets up shop and order from online sources.

"It's Too Expensive"

Yes, sometimes healthier choices are more expensive than what you're used to spending, though that's changing, too. (An increasing number of conventional supermarkets carry grass-fed and organic meats at competitive prices, and local farmer's markets are also an excellent resource.) And remember how expensive flat screens and cell phones used to be? Once consumers made their demands known, the supply rose and the price dropped. It works the same way with a pound of pasture-raised pork.

Cost also depends on what foods you choose. Wild salmon flown in fresh is much more expensive than canned wild salmon, and frozen vegetables are usually cheaper than fresh, yet they have the same nutritional value. If you are on a budget, select products like canned wild salmon and frozen fruits and vegetables.

Think about how much you spend on groceries now and estimate, realistically, how much higher your grocery bill would be if you switched to higher quality foods—a process that you can ease into. The cost may be less than you think, and now that you know the facts about the effect of grain-fed meat on your health, we hope you'll agree that it's worth making a change. The price for cancer therapy can range anywhere from $50,000 to $5 million—now *that* is expensive.

"I Don't Eat That Much Meat or Dairy . . . Why Should I Worry?"

Will two or three servings of conventionally raised meat a week make you sick? Or does it take four or more? We don't know—nor does anyone else. The problem is that once you ingest the toxins in the fat of conventionally raised meat, those poisons will accumulate in your own fat for years, maybe even decades. Before you know it, "just a little" toxic meat every week for a decade could easily result in a huge toxin stockpile.

What we *do* know is that our food is being produced with substances that cause cancer in animals and that have been banned in other developed nations. We also know that omega-6 fats cause inflammation, the basis for disease and weight problems. Why risk eating the old way if you have another option? If you're ready to make a change in how you look and how you feel, then make a change in how you buy your food.

. . . And If You Can't Eat Clean, Eat Lean

We're realistic. You will encounter situations when you can't eat clean—maybe you're traveling and relying on restaurants or your local supplier isn't available. But you need to eat. That's the time to choose *lean* animal protein, such as chicken or turkey breast, pork loin, or beef sirloin. By eating lean you'll avoid most of the stored animal fat, which is the safety deposit box for toxins. Avoid cuts of red meat with lots of fat and avoid all ground beef, which is typically just ground carcass. Or you could avoid meat altogether and have a vegetarian meal—or just go fishing for dinner by choosing some seafood. Our focus has been on land animals, but seafood is an excellent source of mighty omega-3s. As with protein, always choose *clean* seafood, which is most likely to be wild-caught.

THE DOS AND DON'TS OF SMART FAT EGGS AND DAIRY

Finding clearly labeled "grass-fed" and "pasture-raised" meat and poultry is becoming easier, but what about eggs? What about butter, milk, yogurt, and cheese?

Eggs: As of this writing, the availability of eggs from genuinely free-range chickens is not as widespread as that of pasture-raised meat. Unless you are purchasing farm-fresh eggs directly from a local source or raising your own chickens, you may have trouble finding true pastured eggs.

Real free-range chickens on small farms are allowed to live and roam outside, in fresh air, foraging for their food as opposed to being caged and fed. (Industrial egg producers can actually use the "free-range" or "cage-free" label, but this may simply mean that the chickens are not caged; they may still live indoors, in crowded conditions, eating a diet of grain under artificial light. Unlike the label "USDA Certified Organic," no equivalent USDA guidelines for "free-range" are in place to regulate and guarantee consistency.)

Eggs from cage-free, organic-fed chickens are much healthier than conventional eggs, where hens live in tiny cages under filthy conditions and are often sprayed with chemicals just to keep them alive. If you can't find pasture-raised, organic-fed chicken eggs, the cage-free, organic-fed variety in your supermarket are probably an acceptable compromise.

Why not just eat conventional eggs? Because chemicals and hormones are concentrated in the yolk, where the fat is concentrated—in the same way that hormones, pesticides, and other toxins wind up in the fat of conventionally raised meat.

At the very minimum, we recommend you buy organic, cage-free, omega-3-enriched eggs. If you can't get them, then you should avoid eating the yolks, which contain the chemicals concentrated in the fat. You will still get the benefit of the protein, which is concentrated in the egg whites, while you avoid the toxins. Farm-fresh, pasture-raised eggs are the best, in terms of both nutrition and taste. With these kinds of nontoxic eggs, you can eat the yolks to your heart's content.

Butter, Milk, Yogurt, and Cheese: It's increasingly common to find these items from pastured (grass-fed) animals. If you are trying to lose weight through the Smart Fat Solution, you'll see that we don't routinely steer you to reduced-fat or nonfat versions of dairy. We don't recommend nonfat or reduced-fat cheese if it's full of artificial additives to make up for fat that has been removed, but you should look for pastured animal products. At the very minimum, choose organic only. Once again, as with meat, poultry, and eggs, the toxins concentrate in the fat; to avoid toxins, avoid nonorganic products.

Bad Fats That Will Never Be Neutral or Good

We've talked about good, neutral, and bad fats. We want to be clear that bad fats should *always* be on your "do not eat" list.

Trans Fats

Artery-clogging trans fat, which we have likened to embalming fluid that turns our tissues to plastic, is a killer, pure and simple. It's made by combining regular oil with chemicals and harmful metals; then hydrogen is pumped in to solidify the fat—hence the term *hydrogenated* or *partially hydrogenated.* This process also creates a fat that is shelf-stable, a desirable quality for manufacturers of packaged, processed foods. Great for *shelf* life, but not for *your* life.

The invention of hydrogenated and partially hydrogenated fats revolutionized the food industry, specifically, the *junk* food industry, and gave us aisles and aisles of packaged cookies, bread products, cake mixes (and spreadable canned frosting to go with them), crackers, chips, "instant" convenience foods like soups and side dishes, frozen foods, nondairy creamers, microwaveable foods, and much more. Fast-food chains and restaurants loved using trans fats, particularly for frying, because they were cheap and lasted forever.

There was a time when we blamed saturated fats for high levels of "bad" LDL cholesterol. But now we know that trans fats actually raise LDL cholesterol levels, while simultaneously lowering levels of healthy HDL (high-density lipoprotein) cholesterol! Trans fats also elevate your blood sugar and insulin levels and cause a stiffening of the arteries associated with high blood pressure and arterial plaque formation, which leads to deadly cardiovascular disease. In other words: Trans fats will stop your heart. The safe amount of man-made trans fats in the human diet is *zero.* Don't eat them—ever!

Omega-6 Fats

As we've seen, lowering levels of inflammatory omega-6 fats in relation to omega-3 fats is crucial to your health. Products from grain-fed animals are a huge source of omega-6s, but many plant-based oils are also exceedingly high in omega-6.

These are the same oils that have long been marketed to consumers as "heart-healthy" alternatives to animal fats. Corn oil, canola oil, peanut oil, sunflower oil, safflower oil—they literally dominate the cooking oil shelves at the grocery store. Others, like cottonseed and soybean oil, show up in many processed foods. And for decades, we've been told that these are the "good" fats, the ones we should be consuming, while staying away from the "bad" fats, like saturated fat.

It was bad advice.

In 2012, C. E. Ramsden and colleagues analyzed data from the Sydney Diet Heart Study, which divided 458 men with a recent heart attack into two groups. The control group got no specific dietary instruction, but the "intervention" group replaced saturated fat in their diets with vegetable oils. Reanalysis of the data plus analysis of additional previously missing data caused the researchers to come to the unexpected conclusion that substituting these so-called vegetable oils for saturated fat actually increased the risk of death from all causes, including coronary heart disease and cardiovascular disease. "These findings," the researchers wrote, "could have important implications for worldwide dietary advice to substitute omega 6 linoleic acid, or polyunsaturated fats in general, for saturated fats."

There are better alternatives to inflammatory, disease-causing industrial (vegetable) oils. Ignore the "heart-healthy" marketing slogans on the packaging of these generic, processed omega-6–laden oils, because they are anything but heart-healthy.

Chemically Processed "Dirty" Oils

Many of the oils that are high in omega-6s are produced from factory-farmed crops that are heavily sprayed with pesticides and then processed with toxic chemicals and extreme heat, resulting in a highly refined finished product with no nutritional value—about as far from "natural" as possible. Dirty oils are damaged, poisoned fats that are also particularly high in *linoleic acid,* an inflammatory omega-6 fatty acid.

Linoleic acid is an "essential" fatty acid, meaning that it's essential that we get it from our diet since our bodies can't make the stuff. Our bodies need linoleic acid to function, but we don't need a whole lot of it. Unfortunately, most of the omega-6 fats we consume come from these chemically processed industrial seed oils rather than from beneficial whole food sources like nuts and seeds and the cold-pressed organic oils made from them.

The linoleic acid found in these dirty oils contributes to the oxidation of small, dense LDL cholesterol particles, the "bad" cholesterol particles that are the most dangerous because they are involved in the formation of arterial plaque. A high ratio of linoleic acid (omega-6) in relation to omega-3 contributes to heart disease, especially when omega-6s are damaged during chemical processing. At the very least, it certainly contributes to inflammation.

We mentioned above that these bad oils are produced using very high temperatures. Why does that matter? Because when foods containing linoleic acid (omega-6) are exposed to high heat (through processing or through heating up the food itself during cooking), nasty by-products called OXLAMs (oxidized linoleic acid metabolites) are produced. OXLAMs are found in oxidized LDL and in arterial plaque, and they're strongly associated with heart disease; furthermore, high levels of OXLAMs have been found in individuals with Alzheimer's disease, chronic pain, and nonalcoholic steatohepatitis (NASH). NASH is a condition where fat and scar tissue accumulate in the liver; it's like an advanced form of the increasingly common nonalcoholic fatty-liver disease (NAFLD).

A diet *high* in linoleic acid from these refined oils and *low* in beneficial omega-3 fatty acids, such as eicosapentaenoic acid (EPA) and docosahexaenoic acid (DHA), contributes to the inflammation cycle, as well as to the onset of heart disease and other life-threatening conditions. The bottom line: There are no nutritional benefits to eating foods prepared with chemically processed, highly refined dirty oils—no benefits at all, but plenty of risk.

Smart Moves: Trade Your Dumb Fats for Smart Fats

Cut All the Trans Fats

If you want to lose weight, protect your health, and probably extend your life, you should make eliminating all trans fats a top priority. It's not that hard to do. Trans fats are easy to avoid when you know where to look: fried fast foods and other restaurant fare, bags and boxes of prepared convenience foods, packaged baked goods, and virtually anything made with hydrogenated and partially hydrogenated fats. But there's more to ferreting out these toxic fats beyond avoiding the obvious places they lurk.

In recent years, as consumers have gotten wise to the dangers of trans fat, food manufacturers have removed them from many foods (though just because chips are made with "pure sunflower oil" instead of "partially hydrogenated vegetable oil" doesn't make them a good pick). The FDA has ordered their removal from our food supply by 2018, and cities like New York and Philadelphia (not to mention the entire state of California!) have already passed laws that require restaurants to remove most trans fats from their kitchens. McDonald's famously quit cooking their fries in trans fat years ago (yet, just like those chips, that still doesn't make them a healthy food).

But food manufacturers are clever. Through a loophole in the regulations, they're currently allowed to say "zero trans fat" if the product in question has less than one-half gram per serving. By making "serving sizes" unrealistically small, they can claim "zero" trans fat. Meanwhile, you, the consumer, can easily consume a couple of grams in a real-life serving of their product. Multiply this by a few products a day, and before you know it you're consuming trans fat grams in the double digits.

Remember that the ideal daily amount of trans fats in the human diet is zero.

There's one way—and only one way—to tell whether a store-bought item has trans fat in it: *read the label,* specifically the small print of the ingredients list. If you see the words "partially hydrogenated" or "hydrogenated" on the list, it contains trans fat. Put it down and walk away. You've just improved your health.

Restaurants are a tougher challenge. Even in the handful of cities that ban trans fat, the ban is largely still partial, and you can't be 100 percent sure unless you hang out in the kitchen and watch them make your food—or you know the owner *very* well. Ask whether they prepare foods in hydrogenated oils, including hydrogenated soybean oil or a commonly used restaurant product called *phase vegetable oil.* If they do, be thankful that they're being honest and then ask them to please cook your food in olive oil. If they do that (and you trust them), enjoy your meal. If they won't make the change, then don't order it. It's just not worth it. (P.S.: It's time to look for another restaurant.)

Change Your Oil

One of us, Jonny, studied with the renowned late nutritionist Robert Crayhon, who once declared, "If I ever wanted to commit murder and get away with it, all I'd have to do is sneak into a person's kitchen and stock it up with sunflower, safflower, cottonseed, soybean, and corn oil."

It's time to clean out your pantry if you've regularly been buying and using the kinds of poor-quality, refined inflammatory vegetable oils high in omega-6s that we've mentioned. (Just a reminder: There are no vegetables in "vegetable oil"—they are plant-based oils extracted from grains like corn and seeds like safflower.) In the cooking oil section of most supermarkets you'll see nothing but plastic bottle after plastic bottle of low-priced, mass-produced industrial seed and grain oil, and maybe a tiny selection of offbeat oils that you never considered. It's time to start looking closely at what's on those shelves, and what you're putting into your body. (And by the way, choose glass bottles when you purchase oil to avoid toxic chemicals that leach from plastics into oil.)

Here's is a short list of oils to keep in mind when you're shopping. Depending on what you're cooking or baking, or whether you're making a salad dressing, you'll want to choose certain flavors from our "green light" and "yellow light" categories. For instance, with regard to olive oil, extra-virgin olive oil smokes at medium-high heat and changes in composition and flavor, so it's better (and more economical) to save it for salad dressings and for drizzling. Instead, use regular virgin olive oil for cooking at medium-high heat. (See Chapter 10 for more information on smoke points and cooking oils.)

Green Light Oils (Take Them Home): Olive oil, nut oils (almond, walnut, pistachio, macadamia, and pecan), avocado oil, sesame oil, coconut oil, and red palm oil. (If you cook with these, make sure you pick the right oil for the right temperature; see Chapter 10.)

Yellow Light Oils (Slow Down and Look): Peanut oil, canola oil (but *only* organic, glass-bottled, cold-pressed, and expeller-pressed).

Red Light Oils (Stop! Don't Buy): Most of what is sold cheaply in big plastic bottles, like corn oil, "vegetable oil blend," soybean oil.

If you just need some fat to cook with, or are looking for a specific flavor, consider using traditional (animal) fats, but from clean sources only—for instance, organic butter or lard from pasture-raised cows (making a real comeback with serious, health-minded chefs) or fat from pasture-raised ducks. In some markets you can also purchase organic clarified butter, or ghee.

Sugar: The Unsweetened Truth

You already know that eating berry-flavored breakfast cereal that turns the milk pink or guzzling a thirty-two-ounce cola are really lousy ideas. If you're an avid label reader, you're even on to the hoax of that sugar-packed granola bar—a candy bar masquerading as a health food in a grown-up wrapper. If you've been following along, you've connected the dots between eating sugary foods, quick spikes in blood sugar, insulin resistance, glucose conversion, fat cells, inflammation, disease, and, well, death.

So, we won't waste your time and present a list of sugary junk foods that you should avoid. (Hint: If it leaves a powdered sugar residue on your fingers and you bought it at the same place where you filled up your car, then don't eat it.) Those are the obvious, processed carbohydrate foods that should not be a part of a smart fat diet, or *any* diet, unless it's the Get Sick, Die Early Diet.

Instead, let's get back to the less obvious bad guys. Some might say a cinnamon raisin bagel for breakfast is better than a glazed cinnamon bun. Well, maybe, but that's like saying a tornado is better than a hurricane. (You'll see why in a moment.)

Welcome to the Sugar Storm.

The Real Devil in Our Diet

When we first started working on this book, we knew that most people would need some persuading if they were going to change their beliefs about fat. After all, health professionals, government agencies, and health organizations like the American Dietetic Association and the American Heart Association (of which Steven is a member) have been telling people to avoid fat and fill up on "complex carbs" for a very long time. Our telling people to eat fat as a way of getting and staying lean and healthy, particularly after years of hearing "anti-fat" propaganda, goes against the conventional diet "wisdom" of the past several decades. But we went into this knowing that fat—smart fat, that is—was not the bad guy. And the very best medical science backs us up.

Here's the truth: We've been blaming the wrong thing for our epidemic rates of obesity, heart disease, diabetes, and other illnesses that are, in many cases, completely avoidable. The butler didn't do it, and neither did the fat. It was—and is—*sugar,* and all the other hidden forms of *refined carbs.*

In our quest to go low-fat, we stripped our diets of healthy, natural, smart fat. But we didn't just take those fat-based calories out of our diet and end it there. We replaced them with refined carbohydrates. Yes, we successfully avoided many fatty foods, but, as it turns out, we filled the void with foods that were far worse—refined carbohydrate foods that essentially behave in our bodies like spoonfuls of white table sugar, and are only marginally more nutritious. And then we doubled down and replaced saturated fat with inflammatory "vegetable" oils, compounding the problem even further. We suspect by now that we've warned you off of the sugar-coated deep-fried doughball, but let's look at two other sources of the sweet stuff, some of which are frequently presented to us as healthy choices.

1. *Foods Made with Flour*

Breads, pasta, pretzels, crackers, and cereals, made with flour, are technically low in fat and rarely have added sugars (except for many breakfast cereals); but all flours are refined, highly processed carbohydrates. Whether the flour is whole-grain or white, it spikes your blood sugar and insulin levels just the way eating table sugar would, and the metabolic mess that makes us sick and fat happens all over again.

Some people eliminate all foods containing wheat because they have a condition known as *celiac disease.* These folks have horrible reactions to a protein in grains known as *gluten.* But you don't have to have a diagnosis of full-blown celiac to have a bad reaction to gluten, and many people who are gluten-sensitive avoid it for that reason. Other people are less concerned about gluten but simply want to cut back on refined carbohydrates, including flour products, for many of the reasons we've just discussed.

We have a very simple view of products made with flour: Avoid them as much as possible. They will wreck your metabolism, your waistline, your arteries, your brain, and your health.

But isn't whole-grain flour better for you than white flour? Well, yes, but the effects on your blood sugar levels, your metabolism, and your hormones are the same. Whole-grain flour does have slightly more nutrient value than white flour, but the blood sugar response to eating any type of flour product, and the weight gain that goes with it, are why these foods are on our "no fly" list.

2. *Foods with Added Sugar (by Any Name)*

We won't belabor the reasons for cutting out sugary soda and the like—we know you put soda into the same category as that sugar-coated deep-fried doughball. But we do want to point out that added sugar crops up in many foods that are often presented to us as good choices, and it has many aliases.

Let's face it: "Organic cane juice," "maple syrup," and "honey" sound a lot better than "sugar," but they're still sugar, and if it's in your organic (flavored) yogurt, you might as well buy plain yogurt and dump in a few packets of the white stuff. Food manufacturers are required to list ingredients in order of predominance, but they know you'll run the other way if "sugar" is listed first. To get around that, they toss in a couple of sugar sources with other names. Here are some that should trigger an alarm, because we guarantee that if you eat foods containing lots of these substances, your metabolism will quickly be thrown out of whack: glucose, fructose, high-fructose corn syrup (of course), any other kind of syrup (including maple and rice), cornstarch, potato starch, cane products, fruit juice, honey, potato starch, sucrose, and dextrose.

Sugar in these forms can show up in the strangest places, like salty-savory, herb-filled pasta sauces and vinegary dressings—even high-quality ones with organic ingredients. Realistically, you can't keep every molecule of added sugar out of your diet, but because it creeps into your diet more than it should, look at the ingredients—not just the nutrition label—when you're looking for sugar. If you're wondering whether or not artificial sweeteners, or natural sweeteners like

AGAVE NECTAR: HYPE OR HEALTHY?

Agave nectar/syrup is basically high-fructose corn syrup masquerading as a health food. This amber-colored liquid pours more easily than honey and is considerably sweeter than sugar. Its reputation as a health food is based on the fact that it's gluten-free, suitable for vegan diets, *and,* most especially, it's *low glycemic,* meaning that supposedly it has a low effect on blood sugar levels after you ingest it. Largely because of that reason, agave nectar is marketed as "diabetic friendly." What's not to like?

As it turns out, quite a lot.

Agave nectar is considered low glycemic for one reason only: It's largely made of fructose, the sugar found naturally in fruit. Fructose is perfectly fine when you get it from whole foods like apples (which are about 7 percent fructose); in that form, it is packaged with a host of vitamins, antioxidants, and fiber. But when it's commercially extracted from fruit, concentrated, and made into a sweetener, fructose exacts a considerable metabolic price. It may be termed "low glycemic," but we now know that fructose is a very damaging form of sugar when used as a sweetener. Agave nectar has the highest fructose content of any commercial sweetener (with the exception of pure liquid fructose).

All sugar—from table sugar to high-fructose corn syrup (HFCS) to honey—contains *some* mixture of fructose and glucose. Table sugar is 50/50, HFCS is 55/45. But agave nectar is a whopping 90 percent fructose, almost—but not quite—twice as high as HFCS.

Research shows that it's the fructose part of sweeteners that's the most dangerous. Fructose causes insulin resistance and significantly raises triglycerides (a risk factor for heart disease). It also increases fat around your middle, which in turn puts you at greater risk for developing diabetes, heart disease, and Metabolic Syndrome. Fructose has been linked to nonalcoholic fatty-liver disease. Rats given high-fructose diets

CONTINUED ON NEXT PAGE

CONTINUED FROM PAGE 63

develop a number of undesirable metabolic abnormalities, including elevated triglycerides, weight gain, and extra abdominal fat.

In the agave plant, most of the sweetness comes from a particular kind of fructose called *inulin* that does have some health benefits; it's considered a fiber, for one thing. But not much inulin is left in the syrup. During the manufacturing process, enzymes are added to the inulin to break it down into digestible sugar (fructose), resulting in a syrup that has a fructose content that is at best 57 percent and more commonly as high as 90 percent.

Agave nectar syrup is a triumph of marketing over science. (True, it is "low glycemic," but so is gasoline; that doesn't mean it's good for you.) If you're looking for an alternative sweetener, see the information on alternatives to sugar in Chapter 7. Agave is not the answer.

agave nectar, are better than plain old white table sugar, we'll give you the short answer: Not really. (In the case of agave, it's actually much worse; see the box titled "Agave Nectar: Hype or Healthy?") For more information on alternative sweeteners, see Chapter 7.

Perhaps you already knew all those words besides "sugar" that indicate, well, sugar. If so, you're among those savvy consumers who are wise to how unhealthy "healthy" foods can actually be. But even as we're armed with more and more information about our food supply, food producers still try to sell us a constantly updated grocery list packed with sweetened, lightly sweetened, or artificially sweetened products.

In recent years, we've seen a flood of new foods that didn't previously exist but that have been created to meet the demand for more low-fat, low-calorie options. We're talking about beverages like sweetened sports drinks, "juice beverages," sugary flavored waters, even low-fat chocolate milk enriched with omega-3s. Every aisle of the supermarket has sweet "fruit snacks" that hide behind the promise of vitamin C, low-fat yogurts packaged with granola toppings that are nothing more than candy, organic breakfast cereal with just as much sugar as the neon-colored kiddie stuff, 100-calorie packs of cookies (100-calorie packs of everything), and many more deluges from the Sugar Storm.

Don't think that some of these gimmicky foods like squeezable bubble-gum-flavored-yogurt-in-a-tube were cynically created just for kids; adults buy and consume these items, too. (The Centers for Disease Control and Prevention says that men between the ages of twenty and fifty-nine, not kids, are among the biggest consumers of sugar!) And whether or not you can find the word "sugar" on the label, these foods and beverages all have one thing in common: They can ruin your metabolism—and your life.

The Problem with That Cupcake

So how much harm is there in a cupcake, particularly if you bought it at the trendy organic bakery? What's so bad about a scoop of sweet ice cream made with milk from a pasture-raised cow at the local artisanal creamery? Well, the old rationalization "it won't kill you" is probably true, *if* you treat these foods as *treats*.

There are some good reasons behind approaching certain foods, including that dessert made with pasture-raised ingredients, with caution. Specifically, watch out for two sugar combos: (1) sugar and protein, and (2) sugar and fat.

Here's why the dietary combo of sugar and protein is a disaster. Excess sugar is sticky (like cotton candy). Proteins, though, are smooth and slippery, like little tadpoles. This slipperiness is exactly what makes it so easy for proteins to slide around in the cells and do their many jobs effectively.

But when excess sugar keeps bumping into proteins it's like throwing cotton candy in your gas tank. The sugar gums up the works and creates sticky proteins that are too big to get through small blood vessels and capillaries. (That's why diabetics have so many issues with their eyes and feet and kidneys, where many of these tiny vessels hang out.) Eventually, the sugar-coated proteins become toxic, damage the body, and exhaust the immune system. They're also a big factor in aging.

As for sugar and fat, the combination of the two is more lethal than either by itself. You know now that sugar increases inflammation and that inflammation is a major part of just about every modern disease. So, if you eat that artisanal ice cream, even if it's sweetened with organic cane sugar, you've consumed sugar, and on top of it, you've consumed it with fat.

Again, it doesn't really matter whether that ice cream came from a really friendly, clean, pasture-raised cow. When you combine its cream (fat) with sugar, you set off a sharp rise in inflammation. The pastured, organic cream may be a neutral fat, but when fat molecules collide with sugar, inflammation rates increase exponentially; biochemically speaking, it's like a bomb going off in your body. That's bad enough, but think about refined carbohydrate foods like donuts—a lethal combo of truly dumb fat mixed with loads of refined sugar. Welcome to Inflammation Nation.

Other potentially hazardous examples of combined sugar and fats are steak sandwiches, steak and potatoes, cheese and crackers, and pizza (cheese, sausage, and white flour). (If you're thinking that potatoes aren't sugar, think again—they convert to sugar in the body very rapidly.) If once in a while you indulge in a piece of birthday cake— butter and white flour with sugar—it's not the end of the world. (And who among us wants to live in a world where you couldn't have the occasional bowl of premium ice cream?) But if you're eating this stuff daily, watch out! You can avoid the problem by enjoying your grass-fed steak without the bread and potatoes (it's great with a garden-fresh salad) or the organic cheese without the cracker (swap out the cracker and have some luscious slices of fresh pear, instead). These smart choices are much better for your health.

We realize that we've given you a lot of reasons not to eat certain foods—foods that may have been on your list of all-time favorites. So, does all this mean that you can't have a slice of birthday cake with a scoop of ice cream ever again? Of course not.

We're not the Food Police. We're also not Diet Dictators. (The real Diet Dictators are the ones who got us into this mess in the first place.) We are, however, here to share with you what we know about nutrition and health. We know without a doubt that certain foods will short-circuit your health—and shorten your life—and it's our responsibility to let you know that and to show you how smart fats can be the solution.

But we are also realistic. We all have lives. We like to celebrate with friends and family—and food is often a part of that. We have relatives who insist on "doing" Thanksgiving (with the worst trimmings) and a ninety-year-old grandmother who still sends you sugar-cookie care packages. We go on a dream vacation to a city that is famous for its food. A kid is finally home from college and begging to go to a favorite burger joint for a family meal. Your best pal is hosting the annual Super Bowl/Oscars/Memorial Day blowout, and the dining room table is covered with chicken wings, ribs, potato salad, chips and dip, soda, beer—and brownies.

It's up to you to decide whether it's worth it or not.

Your sister's wedding? Special. A midweek lunch with your colleague who likes to get stuffed-crust pizza? Not so special. (But go anyway and use the opportunity to practice your skills by smart-fatting your lunch choice.)

We aren't going to be there with you when you have to make the decision on what to eat and what not to eat. But we are here right now, to give you practical information—and the life-saving science behind it.

CHAPTER 4

Unlearn What You Know About Food

Between the two of us we've met many thousands of people who can reel off calorie counts for hundreds of foods. They also know their total percentage of calories from fat; have memorized total number of grams of protein, saturated fat, and carbs; and can recite these numbers faster than a sports fanatic can rattle off baseball stats. Some of them can even tell you the exact amount of potassium in a potato. In a world in which billions of eaters have access to the Internet, information on food is easy to come by.

Not all that long ago, every conscientious "dieter" had a well-thumbed paperback in the kitchen that listed the calorie counts for everything imaginable. Then the listings got more specific. There were separate books for those who wanted to count carbs and for those who wanted to calculate protein. There were books on how to avoid fat in your diet. Next came books that listed a food's glycemic index. And soon the books themselves were replaced by countless websites and apps for tracking and analyzing every single morsel or sip. Meanwhile, the nutrition and ingredients labels on food packages grew longer and longer—not exactly a good omen for the consumer.

We have a lot of facts at our fingertips about what we eat and drink—more than at any other time in history. But has all this information really helped us? We're still struggling with our weight and our health, diabetes is rampant, we're in the midst of an obesity epidemic, and according to a statistical update from the American Heart Association, heart disease kills almost eight hundred thousand people a year in the United States alone.

Why is this happening?

We have an answer. It may not be the *only* answer—health is, after all, a complex, multidetermined affair—but it's definitely an important *part* of the answer.

We think that one reason for our nutritional dysfunction, and the serious health consequences that have resulted, is because we've learned the wrong lessons from all those facts that we've accumulated about food. We've drawn incorrect or incomplete conclusions; we've misunderstood the science (which is often badly reported, overly hyped, or oversimplified by the media); we've listened to erroneous information from diet and health gurus; and we've been led to believe things that simply aren't true. Sometimes the misinformation is deliberate (like when the facts come from the marketing departments of chemical companies), and sometimes it's innocent (such as advice from well-meaning doctors who just don't know much about nutrition).

Either way, much of the information we've been "taught" has turned out to be dangerous to our well-being. Specifically, we've learned the wrong things about the macronutrients that make up most of our daily diets: carbohydrates, protein, and fat. Now it's time to unlearn what you know about the relationship between these three categories of food and replace it with a real, working knowledge that you can use in a practical way to help you reach your goals. The Smart Fat Solution *will* work for you—for life—and you'll appreciate why once you have all the smart *facts*.

Carbo Load

As you know by now, different kinds of carbohydrates behave differently in your body. Refined carbs, such as white flour and white rice, have virtually the same effect on blood sugar as white table sugar—which is to say, they send your blood sugar on the rollercoaster ride from hell, triggering a cascade of dysfunctional hormonal and metabolic activity. Fiber-rich carbs, however, such as fresh whole vegetables and low-sugar fruits, are a whole different story. These carbs, the kind you could have plucked or gathered if you were a Neanderthal, are a boon to people who want to lose weight. They're equally valuable for anyone who wants to fight inflammation, the silent promoter of nearly every degenerative disease on the planet.

If we know that junky carbs are a metabolic train wreck, then how did we get to a point where they were taking up more than half of our plates? To answer this question, we need to share a little bit of U.S. history—the kind that's known only by nutrition nerds like us.

A Brief History of Dietary Disasters

The 1970s had its low points. And while there are many candidates for the biggest mistake of the decade—Watergate and the AMC Gremlin come to mind—one certainly has to be the first set of dietary guidelines put out by the U.S. government. "Dietary Goals for the United States," prepared by the Select Committee on Nutrition and Human Needs, was very clear in recommending that Americans "increase carbohydrate consumption to account for 55 to 60 percent of the energy (caloric) intake." This championing of carbs came at almost precisely the time in our history that dietary fat was taking a drubbing.

That drubbing, which turned into a full-fledged demonization of fat in all its dietary forms, actually started much earlier, when heart disease was rapidly becoming the leading cause of death in the United States. A noted, and ambitious, physiologist named Ancel Keys had a hunch that this emerging epidemic was somehow related to diet. (As it turns out he was right—but not in the way he believed.)

Keys was a frequent visitor to Italy, where he couldn't help but notice the robust health of the people in the Mediterranean regions, as well as their remarkably low rates of heart disease. He believed that the reason for this was that they ate relatively low amounts of saturated fats. To support this hypothesis, he assembled data on diet and heart disease for male residents from six countries—Japan, Italy, England/Wales, Canada, Australia, and the United States—over a one-year period (1948–1949). Sure enough, he was able to show on a graph that when the men ate a higher percentage of fat calories, they were more likely to die of heart disease. In the 1950s he presented his data to the World Health Organization and was met with quite a bit of skepticism—skepticism that actually turned out to be well-founded.

One of the many problems with Keys's initial graph was that the data didn't come from a study—it was just a carefully chosen collection. Data existed for twenty-two countries, but Keys chose to graph only six. In response to the lack of enthusiasm for his hypothesis, he designed a real study, one of the biggest and most famous studies in all of nutritional epidemiology. Known as the Seven Countries Study, it began in 1958 and lasted nearly twenty years. And—no surprise to anyone—Keys got exactly the results he wanted. The Seven Countries Study, which is cited more often than any other study in nutrition history, did indeed claim to prove that saturated fat is the root cause of heart disease.

Except that it isn't.

Dozens of problems in the Seven Countries Study have emerged since it was first published. For one thing, findings that contradicted Keys's hypothesis were simply ignored. (For example, saturated fat intake was equal on two Greek islands, Crete and Corfu. But the death rate from heart disease was a whopping seventeen times higher on Corfu than on Crete. That difference certainly couldn't be explained by saturated fat intake.) For another, alternate hypotheses were not considered; could something other than saturated fat have accounted for the differences in heart disease rates? Keys dismissed alternatives to the "fat causes heart disease" theory (see, for example, the case of John Yudkin below) because he was convinced that his theory was right.

And that's the kiss of death for real objective science.

At about the same time that Keys was promoting his theory, British physician and researcher John Yudkin was also wondering about the increase in heart disease in First World countries. But Yudkin suggested a different culprit. He pointed out in a series of papers that sugar consumption had a stronger relationship to heart disease mortality than fat did. Keys, however, ignored these inconvenient facts and instead slammed Yudkin in the press at every opportunity. Eventually, as an influential member of the nutrition advisory committee to the American Heart Association, Keys managed to get his theories officially incorporated into the 1961 American Heart Association dietary guidelines. For decades, the American Heart Association has exerted a powerful influence on government health recommendations regarding heart disease, cholesterol, and fat consumption.

The message that *eating fat makes you fat*—and leads you on an irreversible path to heart disease—was not lost on the American people, and the notion that fat is "bad" has become nothing less than a cultural meme.

What's interesting is that the conventional wisdom on fat in the diet was very different before Keys and the Seven Countries Study. Before Keys's theories became entrenched, most doctors knew that the cause of obesity was sugar and starch, not dietary fat. William Osler, known as the father of modern medicine in North America, suggested that people should "reduce sugar and starches" to avoid obesity as early as 1892 in his classic textbook *The Principles and Practice of*

Medicine. Dr. Richard Mackarness, who ran Britain's first obesity and food allergy clinic, wrote in 1958 that carbohydrates were the culprit in weight gain in his book *Eat Fat and Grow Slim.*

But what got everyone's attention was when President Dwight D. Eisenhower suffered a heart attack in 1955. This created a huge interest in what was coming to be understood as the No. 1 killer of men *and* women—heart disease. Eisenhower's attack made the danger real for a lot of people, and Americans wanted answers about this new threat to their health. And they wanted them *now.* The government was pressured to take action and make some dietary recommendations. Waiting for more conclusive science was just not an option.

In the face of such pressure, the government and numerous health organizations and healthcare providers fell in line behind the American Heart Association recommendations, which included Keys's theories. Americans, who wanted to know what they could do to beat this killer, got their official answer: Avoid fat and eat lots of "complex carbohydrates."

Unfortunately, this was the wrong answer.

We know now that Keys's conclusion was incorrect. But his overall message caught on; the anti-fat revolution was born; and the high-carb, low-fat diet and lifestyle took hold—ultimately resulting in an epidemic of obesity, disease, and accelerated aging that still has us in its grip.

You may notice that we're suddenly talking a lot about fat, though we started out focusing on carbs. That's because you can't discuss the damage that refined carbohydrates can do without talking about the role of dietary fat. After all, there are only three macronutrients—protein, fat, and carbohydrates. If you eat less of one of them, you wind up eating more of the others. In our case, we stripped beneficial smart fat from our diets and replaced it with the worst type of carbs—mostly the kind that come in a box. And we've been doing that for about four decades, all in the name of good health.

It hasn't worked out so well.

Removing smart fat from our diets was hardly the only thing we collectively did to raise the risk of heart disease and obesity. Smoking, for instance, used to be widely accepted behavior. In fact, the emerging epidemic of heart disease was occurring at a time when even *physicians* routinely endorsed cigarettes. ("More doctors smoke Camels than any other cigarette!") And while we puffed away, food manufacturers were beginning to add something quite deadly to our diets: trans fats.

In midcentury America, the "Crisco Creep" was in full-swing, with home cooks, food manufacturers, and even the American Heart Association embracing the use of highly engineered dumb fats like margarine and hydrogenated (and partially hydrogenated) "vegetable" oils. For home cooks and dieters trying to do the right thing, these artificial fats seemed like the answer because they were increasingly presented as heart-healthy alternatives to saturated animal fats like butter and lard. For big food companies, hydrogenated fats allowed for the mass production of shelf-stable baked goods, snack foods, convenience foods, and fast food—profitable, booming business sectors that were rapidly growing in postwar America. Trans fats were in the right place at the right time.

So was high-fructose corn syrup. Though arguably no worse than regular sugar, it was spectacularly cheaper. Food manufacturers began adding it to everything, partially to compensate for how bad foods taste when you take out the fat. The wide availability and ubiquity of high-fructose corn syrup partially accounts for the fact that between the 1950s and 2000, per capita consumption of caloric sweeteners increased 39 percent to an average of a whopping 152 pounds per person per year.

And let's not forget another critical factor. While all this was happening—the banishment of fat from our diets, our increased intake of processed carbohydrates, and our reliance on dumb fats like margarine—we were becoming less physically active. After World War II, we rapidly became a car culture and no longer went everywhere (some might say *any*where) on foot. We went from working the land to working the phone. Kids didn't get to school on two wheels or two feet; they got a ride. Sidewalks were sacrificed for wider roads to accommodate more cars. We had lots of new reasons to be sedentary. (The postwar Golden Age of Television was only the beginning of our love affair with the screen.) We no longer experienced exercise as something built in to our days. Instead, we had to schedule a "workout," and who could possibly make time for that?

So there you have it. We began reducing naturally occurring dietary fat to avoid heart disease, even though recent evidence shows no connection between fat in the diet—even *saturated* fat—and heart disease; simultaneously, we increased our consumption of toxic trans fats and refined carbohydrates, all the while decreasing our level of physical activity. Our food supply became more industrialized (and toxic) as factory-farmed meat from huge agricultural feedlot operations replaced grass-fed cattle, free-range chickens, and pasture-raised pigs. Before factory farms became the norm, it was easy to follow our prescription to eat clean, not mean.

Within one generation, out went the farm-fresh eggs and bacon and in came the breakfast of sugary cereal, white-bread toast slathered with margarine, and, of course, a glass of sweet orange juice—the ultimate "low-fat" (and therefore "healthy") breakfast. Gone was the home-cooked dinner of roasted chicken and garden-fresh vegetables, replaced by chemically laden mystery meat, a few scoops of starch, and a tiny mound of overcooked mixed vegetables. And in between that breakfast and dinner was a lunch break that increasingly involved another dining trend, one that was rapidly becoming an everyday habit for millions: fast food. (But even dinner quickly became fast food. That wholesome, homemade roasted chicken dinner eventually became a bucket of chicken pieces from the drive-through, a side of creamed corn, biscuits, and a liter of soda.)

Our new diet—low in fat, high in refined carbs, and meant to rescue us from heart disease—was actually killing us. Here's why.

The Coming of the Plague:
The Rise of Metabolic Syndrome

If your goal is weight loss, you'll be successful if you follow the Smart Fat Solution. But that weight loss is just a wonderful side effect of something even *more* beneficial, *and* life-saving: protection against what we call the Black Plague of the twenty-first century—Metabolic Syndrome.

Metabolic Syndrome, which we believe is *the* primary cause of heart disease, is actually a collection of risk factors for heart disease and diabetes (it's also known as Syndrome X, prediabetes, or, more recently, "diabesity"). People with Metabolic Syndrome are twice as likely to die from heart disease—and three times more likely to have a heart attack or stroke—than people without it. They have a fivefold greater risk of developing type 2 diabetes, and up to 80 percent of the two hundred million people with diabetes globally will eventually die of cardiovascular disease. Metabolic Syndrome is serious stuff—so much so that the International Diabetes Federation considers it a "global time bomb." And from a healthcare perspective, we spend 500 percent more money on medical care for people with Metabolic Syndrome than for healthy people without it.

So, what exactly *is* Metabolic Syndrome? It's a group of risk factors that taken together hugely increase the risk for developing heart disease, obesity, and diabetes. And what makes it all the more insidious is that many of the risk factors for Metabolic Syndrome have no symptoms, at least not until severe damage has been done.

If you've got three or more of these conditions, then according to the American Heart Association, you've got Metabolic Syndrome. (And by our standards, having even one or two of them translates into accelerated aging). We'll get into a more detailed discussion of these conditions in a moment, but chances are, if you have even one of them, you're on the way to developing another . . . and then another . . . and then another.

It's estimated that 30 percent of all adults and 50 percent of baby boomers have Metabolic Syndrome, but we estimate that two out of three people—even those who appear to be healthy—are walking around with some combination of these lethal risk factors:

- Expanding waistline (for men, more than 40 inches; for women, more than 35)
- Elevated blood pressure (higher than 130/85 mm Hg)
- High triglycerides (higher than 150 mg/dL)
- Low HDL cholesterol (lower than 40 mg/dL in men; lower than 50 mg/dL in women)
- Inflammation (as measured by a high rate of elevated C-reactive protein)[†]
- High fasting blood sugar (higher than 100 mg/dL). (Note: Surprisingly, high blood sugar levels are often the last sign to occur, even though Metabolic Syndrome is often called prediabetes. The scary thing is that many people with Metabolic Syndrome will die from it *before* their blood sugar levels become elevated.)

The take-home point here is that every one of these factors indicates *increased risk for disease and accelerated aging.* And all of them are all directly affected by eating too many refined carbohydrates.

Let's start with triglycerides, the main form of fat in the diet and in the body. Diets that are high in refined carbs greatly increase the likelihood that blood sugar will be elevated, and when that happens, high levels of triglycerides almost always result. (Conventional lab tests define "high" triglycerides as anything higher than 150 mg/dL, but we think anything higher than 100 mg/dL is too high.) If you have high triglycerides, you have a higher risk of arterial plaque growth. Eating refined carbohydrates is the surest way to raise your triglycerides— and a diet lower in refined carbs is the surest way to drop them.

HDL cholesterol is the good guy, head of the clean-up crew, the "garbage collector" who travels through your bloodstream and picks

---

[†] Conventional medicine does not include inflammation as one of the markers of Metabolic Syndrome, but we feel it's clinically important and worthy of inclusion as one of the risk factors.

up all the trashy remnants of damaged LDL cholesterol. You want HDL levels to be high, not low—"ideally" higher than 50 mg/dL for men and 60 mg/dL for women.

But there's much more to the cholesterol story than the old-fashioned division between "good" (HDL) and "bad" (LDL) cholesterol. We now know that there are different types of both HDL cholesterol (for example, HDL-2 and HDL-3) and LDL cholesterol (LDL-a and LDL-b), and they act quite differently in the body. More important than just your overall cholesterol numbers are the *size and number* of the cholesterol particles themselves, regardless of whether those particles are found in HDL or LDL cholesterol. In general, big fluffy molecules of cholesterol don't do any damage, while small dense ones do. A diet high in refined carbs and bad fats will raise the number of small, dense, athrogenic (those that form artery plaque) cholesterol particles and lower the number of big fluffy harmless ones. A diet lower in sugar and processed carbs has the exact opposite effect.

Simply put, the risk factors for Metabolic Syndrome are connected

A NUMBER WORTH KNOWING: YOUR RATIO OF TRIGLYCERIDES TO HDL CHOLESTEROL

The ratio of your triglycerides to HDL cholesterol is an excellent indicator of heart health. It's also an excellent marker for insulin resistance (or its opposite, insulin sensitivity). You want this ratio to be low—2 or less is wonderful. When it's high, it's cause for concern, or even better, action. (You'll find both of these numbers on the results of your routine blood work, or you can calculate this ratio yourself; see our website at www. SmartFat.com for instructions, or ask your healthcare provider.)

You can easily drop your triglycerides (a risk factor for heart disease) when you follow the Smart Fat Solution Thirty-Day Plan (see Chapter 6), which will immediately improve your ratio of triglycerides to HDL cholesterol as well.

by diet. Consuming too many carbohydrates and bad fats will set up the conditions for this dangerous constellation of factors, but because of its combination of fats, protein, and fiber (the *right* carbs), the Smart Fat Solution is a powerful protector against every one of them.

The Carb Conundrum: Why It's Easy to Choose the Wrong Ones

It's easy to spot the junky carbs, but trickier to spot the junk masquerading as health food. As we have already mentioned, some carbohydrate foods that are considered to be healthy, such as whole-wheat bagels, deserve a second look. Just because something is made with a whole grain, is it healthy? The short answer? No.

There are also some carbohydrate foods that definitely are *not* junk. We're talking about fiber-rich, nutrient-packed fruits and vegetables— and as you know, fiber is an essential part of the Smart Fat Solution. Fruits and vegetables are healthy sources of fiber, but these two categories of plant foods, which are often lumped together as equally beneficial, can be quite different in terms of how they affect your body.

Let's take a closer look at some carbs that cause confusion. Grains, the first category, especially deserve more scrutiny before they make it onto our plates.

"Whole" Grains and Half-Truths

As part of the war on heart disease (and by default, the war on Metabolic Syndrome), the Diet Dictators frequently point to one particular weapon of choice: healthy whole grains. This trend started decades ago when suddenly, it seemed, wheat bread began replacing white bread in kitchens across the United States. A brownish bagel with a little shower of oats on top was a "healthy" choice. Cereal made with whole grains, even if those grains were coated with added sugar, was in the bowl every morning. (Unfortunately, it still is.) Big Food has now given us aisles and aisles of whole-grain "alternatives" to bleached grains—just take a look at the typical supermarket's collection of "whole-grain" tortilla chips and pretzels. Then, they tossed "multigrain" into the mix, which somehow seemed even healthier—at

THE WHOLE (GRAIN) TRUTH
AND NOTHING BUT THE TRUTH

Grains can be real troublemakers—especially wheat. You now know how grains, including whole grains, can set off blood sugar fluctuations and the metabolic problems associated with them. There is also the issue of gluten (see Chapter 7 for more on gluten) for the 20 percent of the population who cannot tolerate gluten.

However, some grains are nutrient-dense foods that anyone can enjoy who doesn't have a gluten issue or who is not affected by the blood sugar changes triggered by grains.

- Steel-cut oats
- Quinoa (it's actually a seed, but it looks and cooks like a grain)
- Wild rice
- Brown rice

Note that white rice does not make the cut; it converts quickly to sugar and doesn't provide any nutrients. We also don't include barley. Although it is a low-glycemic grain, it contains gluten, which is problematic for anyone avoiding gluten. Polenta is an increasingly popular food, but it's made from corn, which is very high-glycemic.

One option for slowing down the sugar payload of grains is to combine them with other ingredients, including smart fat. For instance, instead of just plain quinoa or wild rice, make a salad or side dish by combining the grains with loads of fresh or sautéed vegetables, topped with some toasted walnuts and a bit of crumbled goat cheese. Have this as part of a meal that includes a serving of clean protein, and you'll change how the grain affects your body, both inside and out.

least if you could ignore the fact that 80 percent of multigrain foods are made mostly with white flour and have only a few whole grains sprinkled in. At the end of the day, are all these foods really any better than the same products made with white flour?

Actually, no. They're not.

Whole-grain flour contains more nutrients and fiber than white flour. But it has the *same* effect on your blood sugar: It elevates it very quickly. All grains were originally whole grains (so "made from whole grains" is kind of meaningless on a label). But once that grain is ground into flour, it behaves very much like white table sugar in your body.

If you're still thinking that a whole-grain cracker has got to be a better choice than a regular one, just look closely at the ingredients list. It may have some variety of "whole" grain listed, but whether it's a cracker, a slice of bread, a bagel, or pasta, it also contains some form of *ground* grains, or maybe "enriched" flour. That's got to be good for you, right? After all—it's enriched with vitamins!

Well, think for a minute. Why do food manufacturers have to enrich that bread in the first place? Because when they ground the grain (organic or not) into flour, they removed anything that *might* have been good for you. In order to process the grain into shelf-stable flour for that loaf of bread, box of cereal, cracker, or dried pasta, they removed the germ (because it contains an oil that would go rancid) and the bran (there goes the fiber) and then pulverized the life out of the remaining endosperm—essentially stripping this plant food of any nutritional value. Once ground and no longer whole, refined and totally ruined, grains become worthless (and harmful) white flour, empty calories not worth eating. The fact is that commercially manufactured "whole-grain" products generally contain some amount of plain old flour.

We've been told that eating whole grains is the way to go—they're one of the pillars of low-fat, high-carb eating and are often held up as ideal sources of fiber. But here's the truth: Unless you're standing in an organic wheat field and eating the whole grains right off the stalk to get some fiber, you're not eating 100 percent healthy whole grains. There are better, tastier, and more versatile ways to increase your fiber (and we tell you about them in the next chapter). Don't buy the myth that you need to rely on whole grains to get your fiber.

Remember that when grain is turned into flour—white or wheat—it acts like any refined carbohydrate in your body, causing that inflammatory spike in blood sugar. Whether you're eating a whole-grain tortilla or a slice of white bread, the result is the same—it's bad.

Fruits and Vegetables

Fruits and vegetables are both considered "good" carbohydrates and have been lumped together as equal partners for decades. But they can have somewhat different effects on the body, especially when processed.

A few years ago, the USDA replaced the once-vaunted "food guide pyramid" with a new graphic of a plate of food, showing half of it filled with fruits and vegetables (with vegetables, admittedly, taking up slightly more real estate, but not by much). The USDA's 2010 dietary guidelines had suggested a general "five servings a day" of fruits and vegetables, once again making the two categories seem equal.

"Eat more! Fill half your plate with fruits and veggies!" was the official tagline for the "Fruit & Veggies—More Matters" campaign that was kicked off in conjunction with the new "MyPlate" graphic. (Note: This campaign was, and still is, underwritten in large part by grocery stores, produce growers and distributors, and other businesses that have a vested interest in upping produce sales—and their involvement may also explain why fruit juice "counts" as a fruit in some literature.)

Now, you've probably known since you were a kid that these two categories of foods are different. Just ask yourself which you liked better: grapes or green beans. Chances are you liked grapes better—and for an understandable reason. They were sweeter.

Most vegetables have a negligible effect on blood sugar—some, like broccoli, actually have *none*. That's why, from our point of view, they're an *unlimited* food (the exceptions being superstarchy veggies like white potatoes, which quickly convert to sugar). Nonstarchy vegetables (and even a few starchy ones, like peas) are rich in fiber and nutrients, so enjoy.

Sweet-tasting fruits, however, generally have a much higher effect on blood sugar levels than vegetables because of their naturally occurring sugar content. There are also some significant calorie differences between a cup of kale and a cup of mango, if you're concerned about calories. These are the reasons why we ask you to be mindful about your fruits and vegetables.

Here are some of our favorite low-sugar fruits:

- Berries (strawberries, blackberries, blueberries, raspberries)
- Grapefruit
- Apples
- Watermelon
- Cherries
- Pears
- Kiwi
- Peaches
- Cantaloupe
- Oranges

Some fruits, like dried fruits, ripe bananas, and papaya, have very concentrated levels of sugars, so we ask you to avoid them—as well as fruit juices—altogether. (For more on why we think it's time to break the glass-of-juice-with-breakfast habit, see Chapter 7.) They're okay for an occasional treat, but be aware that they can spike blood sugar like a piece of candy does—though of course they offer nutrients that candy doesn't have. If you are trying to break out of insulin and leptin resistance, steer clear. Instead, opt for whole, raw fruits for more fiber and nutrients—and don't forget to eat your veggies!

So what's the final word on fruits and whole grains? We're certainly not saying that you should never eat them. Most fruits, for example, in their whole, unprocessed state, are marvelous foods. But there is simply no getting around the fact that some forms of fruit (such as fruit juice and fruit "leather") and most grains behave in your body exactly like the high-carb foods that they are, sending your blood sugar levels up and triggering that metabolic waltz you know so well by now.

There is, however, a way out of the carb confusion, if you're trying to tell the good from the bad. The key to avoiding Metabolic Syndrome is choosing foods that don't ruin your blood sugar levels.

A *Really* Smart Move: Using Glycemic Load to Help You Choose the Right Carbohydrate Foods

The *glycemic index* is a measure of how quickly and how high your blood sugar rises after eating food. But it's not nearly as important as a less famous measure called the *glycemic load.*

Let's review what we said earlier regarding blood sugar and insulin, and you'll see why the glycemic load matters to your health.

When we eat any food, especially carbohydrates and to some extent proteins, our blood sugar goes up. (It hardly goes up at all when we eat fat.) In response to the rise in blood sugar, our pancreas secretes the hormone insulin, which directs the excess sugar out of the bloodstream and into the cells where, ideally, it can be used for fuel. Blood sugar (and insulin) both gradually go back down to the levels before we ate anything, and in a few hours our bodies repeat the process when we eat again.

When we overeat high-sugar carbohydrates, we quickly drive our blood sugar up into the stratosphere. The pancreas sends out increasing amounts of insulin in an attempt to lower that spike. Unfortunately, if we are sedentary (as too many of us are), our muscle cells aren't interested in answering insulin's call. Insulin knocks on the doors of the muscle cell walls, and the cells say, "Sorry, we don't need any sugar for fuel because our guy's going to be sitting at the computer all day (again), so go somewhere else." So the sugar winds up going to the fat cells, which are far more welcoming. Meanwhile, both blood sugar and insulin have been raised, setting you up for hypertension, fat storage, hunger, cravings, and mood crashes when your sugar eventually does fall—not a great situation. (If you want to review this process in detail, see Chapter 2 where we discuss insulin, cortisol, and leptin.)

Glycemic Index vs. Glycemic Load

To measure the effect of food on blood sugar, scientists came up with the idea of the glycemic index for foods, which you can easily find online—this information is nearly as ubiquitous as calorie counts. Using pure glucose (glycemic index = 100) as the standard, they tested 50-gram portions of digestible carbohydrate and measured how quickly and how high blood sugar rose in reaction to eating these foods. By eating foods with a low glycemic index, you presumably could avoid the blood sugar roller coaster. (Food manufacturers have jumped on the index as a selling point, marketing it on some packaged foods with an official-looking seal hollering "LOW G.I."; but they are often misrepresenting the effect that food will have on your blood sugar. Read on.)

There are two big problems with using the glycemic index as a guide to eating. First of all, the index is designed to measure how quickly and how high your blood sugar rises in response to a fixed quantity (50 grams) of carbohydrates. When it comes to blood sugar, portion size is very important. Let's look at two foods that illustrate this point well: spaghetti, which rates as a "moderate" glycemic index food, and carrots, which rate as a "high" one.

The glycemic index of spaghetti may be "moderate," but no one eats only 50 grams of spaghetti. Why? Because that's only 1 cup, cooked. That's not-a-lotta pasta, and few diners tuck into a single cup of spaghetti and are satisfied. A person is more likely to eat something like 2 cups (and typically much more), which at the very least doubles the index. A real-world serving of spaghetti isn't "moderate" at all in terms of what it does to your blood sugar—it's *high*. As for carrots, 50 grams of carrots translates into nine big carrots. Have you ever eaten nine whole carrots in one sitting? Would you want to try? Because that's what you'd have to do—and you'd have to eat them in a matter of minutes, like a rabbit or a horse—to send your blood sugar rocketing to a high level. Carrots, which people have been known to avoid as a "bad" food because of its "high" glycemic index, have very low glycemic effects, as do most vegetables (most have none whatsoever).

The second problem with using glycemic index as a guide to eating is that these measurements are based on what happens when the food is eaten alone—not with other foods that could affect (that is, slow down) the rate at which blood sugar rises. A banana eaten with peanut butter (a neutral fat) has a slower release in your system than a banana eaten alone. (And instead of half a cup of plain pasta, have that same portion but tossed with white beans and pesto, with a serving of fish or chicken, and you have a much better blood sugar—and dining—experience.)

And the Winner Is . . .

To get a more accurate measure than the glycemic index, food scientists started calculating something called the *glycemic load* (GL), which tells you what's going to happen to your blood sugar when you eat a real-life portion of the food in question. Who cares what the glycemic index is when it's based on a portion size that may have nothing to do with reality? What you want to know is what a *real-life* portion is going to do to your blood sugar, and that's exactly what the GL does. That's why we recommend paying attention to it instead of the glycemic index.

GL data are not as trendy or perhaps as comprehensive for some food categories as the glycemic index, but they are becoming easier to find. You'll find several resources online, including

- The University of Sydney (Australia); http://www.glycemicindex .com/foodSearch.php
- Self NutritionData; http://nutritiondata.self.com/

We've put together a general chart to give you a framework for gauging low-, medium-, and high-GL foods. This information is not comprehensive (which is why we recommend the resources above), but it's designed to show you how some major categories of foods (such as grains and flour products) are considered high-GL, while others (virtually all vegetables, except potatoes) have no GL to speak of.

The GL is not the only way to judge food, but it's an important indicator when you're trying to make sense of carbohydrates and their relationship to fat, fiber, and protein—particularly if you're trying to lose weight.

GLYCEMIC LOAD (GL) OF COMMON FOODS		
Key: 0-9 = low GL; 10-19 = medium GL; 20+ = high GL. Note: Numbers may vary by a few points from one reference to another.		
FOOD	SERVING SIZE	GLYCEMIC LOAD (per serving)
BAKERY PRODUCTS		
MEDIUM GL		
Corn tortilla	50 g (2 tortillas)	12
Flour tortilla	50 g (1 tortilla)	15
Pumpernickel bread	2 slices	13
Vanilla wafers	6 cookies (1 oz)	14
Rice cakes	1 oz	18
Kaiser roll	1 roll (1 oz)	12
Hamburger bun	2 slices	18
Cupcake, strawberry icing	1 cupcake	19
HIGH GL		
Whole-wheat bread	2 slices	20
Wonder Bread	2 slices (2 oz)	20
Donut, glazed	One 4-in diameter	22
Chocolate cake with icing	⅙th cake, 84 g	25
Bagel, white	3.5-in bagel	34

FOOD	SERVING SIZE	GLYCEMIC LOAD
BEVERAGES		
LOW GL		
Unsweetened tea and coffee	1 cup	0
Tomato juice (canned)	1 cup	4
Skim milk	1 cup	9
Whole milk	1 cup	9
Soy milk	1 cup	9
MEDIUM GL		
Apple juice (unsweetened)	1 cup	12
Gatorade	1 cup	12
Orange juice (unsweetened)	1 cup	12
HIGH GL		
Cranberry juice cocktail (Ocean Spray)	1 cup	24
Coca Cola	12-oz can	25
Fanta (orange soda)	12-oz can	35
CEREALS		
LOW GL		
Steel-cut oatmeal	1 cup	9
MEDIUM GL		
Oatmeal, rolled	1 cup	13
Cheerios	1 cup	13
Grits, cooked	1 cup	14
Instant oatmeal	1 cup	16
All-Bran cereal (Kellogg's)	1 cup	16
Grape-Nuts	1 cup	16
Muesli (oats, nuts, dried fruit)	1 cup	16
Special K	1 cup	14
Kashi Go Lean Crunch	1 cup	17
HIGH GL		
Coco Pops	1 cup	20
Corn flakes	1 cup	24
Raisin Bran (Kellogg's)	1 cup	26
Granola (Kashi)	1 cup	37
GRAINS		
MEDIUM GL		
Pearled barley, cooked (has gluten)	1 cup	11
Wild rice, cooked	1 cup	16

FOOD	SERVING SIZE	GLYCEMIC LOAD
Quinoa, cooked	1 cup	18
Spaghetti, whole-meal, boiled	1 cup	15
HIGH GL		
Brown rice, medium-grain, cooked	1 cup	22
Sweet corn	1 cup	22
Spaghetti, white, boiled 10 min	1 cup	22
Macaroni (elbow), cooked	1 cup	23
Macaroni and cheese (Kraft)	1 cup	32
White rice, long-grain, cooked	1 cup	27
White basmati rice, quick-cooking	1 cup	28
Couscous, boiled 5 min	1 cup	30
COOKIES, SNACKS, CRACKERS, CHIPS		
LOW GL		
Hummus (chickpea salad dip)	30 g	0
Guacamole	¼ cup	0
Dark chocolate (70%–85% cocoa)	1 oz	4
MEDIUM GL		
Popcorn, popped	2 cups	12
Oatmeal cookies	1.5 oz	18
Ginger snap cookies	1 oz	17
Granola bar	2-oz bar	18
HIGH GL		
Ginger snap cookies	1.5 oz	24
Nachos, tortilla chips, salted	3-oz bag	35
Pretzels, oven-baked	2-oz bag	33
Mars bar	2-oz bar	27
Potato chips	4-oz bag	30
DAIRY		
MEDIUM GL		
Plain low-fat Greek yogurt	245 g	10
Reduced-fat yogurt with fruit	200 g	11
HIGH GL		
Ice cream, regular	1 cup	24
FRUITS		
LOW GL		
Apple	1 medium	6
Apricots	1 cup	6

FOOD	SERVING SIZE	GLYCEMIC LOAD
Blueberries, wild	1 cup	1
Blueberries, commercially raised	1 cup	4
Cherries	1 cup	4
Grapes	1 cup	5
Grapefruit	1 small	3
Mango	1 cup (120 g)	8
Orange	1 medium	4
Peach	1 large	5
Pear	1 medium	5
Pineapple	1 cup	7
Plums	1 cup	5
Strawberries	1 cup	3
Watermelon	1 cup	4
MEDIUM GL		
Apricot, dried	¼ cup	10
Banana, regular (yellow without spots)	1 medium	10
Banana, ripe (brownish with many spots)	1 medium	16
Dates, dried	¼ cup	14
Fruit juice	1 cup	12
Papaya	1 cup	10
Prunes	¼ cup	14
Raisins	¼ cup	18
BEANS		
LOW GL		
Black beans	½ cup	7
Chickpeas	½ cup	8
Navy beans	½ cup	7
Kidney beans	½ cup	7
Lentils	½ cup	6
Soybeans (edamame)	½ cup	3
White beans	½ cup	9
MEDIUM GL		
Baked beans	½ cup	10
NUTS (dry-roasted) 1 oz = 1 handful		
ONLY LOW GL		
Almonds	1 oz	0
Hazelnuts	1 oz	0

FOOD	SERVING SIZE	GLYCEMIC LOAD
Macadamia nuts	1 oz	0
Pecans	1 oz	0
Pistachios	1 oz	0
Walnuts	1 oz	0
Peanuts (actually a legume)	1 oz	0
Cashews, salted	1 oz	3
VEGETABLES		
LOW GL		
Artichoke (Jerusalem)	1 cup	0
Asparagus	1 cup	3
Avocado (Florida or California fruit)	½ fruit	0
Beets	1 cup	6
Bok choy	1 cup	0
Broccoli	1 cup	0
Cabbage	1 cup	0
Carrots	1 cup	2
Cauliflower	1 cup	0
Celery	1 cup	0
Mixed greens, lettuce, and raw spinach	1 cup	0
Peas, frozen or fresh	1 cup	5
Green bell pepper	1 cup	2
Red or yellow bell pepper	1 cup	3
Parsnip	1 cup	8
MEDIUM GL		
Sweet potato	1 medium (½ cup)	10
Potato salad	1 cup	13
Boiled white and purple potatoes	1 cup	14
Instant mashed potatoes	1 cup	17
HIGH GL		
Baked russet potato	1 medium (5 oz)	26
ANIMAL PROTEIN AND SMART FAT		
LOW GL		
Steak, chicken, salmon, pork	6 oz	0
Eggs	2 eggs	0
Olive, nut, and coconut oil	1 Tbsp	0
Avocado (Florida or California fruit)	½ fruit	0

FOOD	SERVING SIZE	GLYCEMIC LOAD
ALCOHOLIC BEVERAGES		
LOW GL		
Red or white wine	5 oz	0
Vodka	1.5 oz	0
Beer	12 oz	3

A few takeaways to note, before we move to our next chapter and put this information to work:

Most breakfast cereals are medium- or high-GL. On occasion, that's not necessarily a bad thing, but consider what most Americans believe is a "healthy" breakfast: cold cereal with milk, orange juice, and toast. The cumulative glycemic impact of such a breakfast is a GL of at least 49.5, which is a metabolic disaster—all medium- to high-glycemic foods that are pretty much guaranteed to raise your blood sugar too high and leave you hungry an hour later. Keep in mind: What you need in the morning for health and weight control to optimize your hormones is protein, fiber, smart fat, and hydration. The last thing you want first thing in the morning is a big load of sugar. (A better choice is a Smart Fat Shake or any of the breakfast ideas you'll find in Chapter 10.)

The method of food preparation matters. Regular spaghetti boiled until it is very soft (more than twelve minutes; in restaurants where it's not made to order, it often boils for twenty minutes and then sits) has a higher GL than whole-grain spaghetti cooked for a shorter amount of time and served al dente.

Density matters. When eating flour products, the denser the flour, the lower the GL. That's why bread (light and fluffy) compared with rice has a higher GL, and rice has a higher GL than pasta, which is denser.

All vegetables are low-GL. As we pointed out in our discussion of fruits and vegetables, fruits are terrific and are mainly low-GL (except for bananas and papayas—and fruit juice), but they have more sugar than the average vegetable (except for potatoes). Vegetables won't affect your blood sugar, but they will deliver fiber and loads of nutrients.

No grains are low-GL. Except for steel-cut oats, most grains are moderate- to high-GL, so it's best to eat small portions.

All smart fats and protein foods are naturally low-GL. We don't include many fats and proteins in our chart because our focus here is on helping you choose your carbs wisely, but their low GL makes them a great complement to the rest of your smart fat diet.

Here's the science lesson: Eating medium- to high-GL foods increases sugar surges, insulin spikes, insulin resistance, and leptin resistance. If you want to unblock insulin and leptin resistance, steering clear of medium-GL and especially high-GL foods is the way to go. Once your insulin and leptin responses normalize, you can have medium-GL foods from time to time, but watch portion size (and stay away from high-GL foods or you'll "break" your insulin function all over again!).

And here's the practical application of this lesson: Eat as little sugar as possible, and go easy on the foods that turn into sugar quickly, such as cereals, breads, pasta, and other flour products.

Think of the glycemic load as your personal "carb compass"—a way to make smart choices so that the Smart Fat Solution works most effectively.

PART TWO

Smart-Fat Your Food

CHAPTER 5

The Smart Fat Solution

W E KNOW YOU'RE LOOKING FOR A CHANGE—and not just a temporary fix that will last for a few weeks or months or for the length of the two-phase Thirty-Day Plan that you'll find in the next chapter—but big, lasting, and positive change for lifelong good health, including meeting your weight-loss goals and feeling healthier and stronger than ever. It's time to get started and find your Smart Fat Solution.

You know the reasons why we advocate smart fats, protein, and fiber. We've given you the science behind our message (and if you're hungry for more facts, visit our website, www.SmartFat.com, for the latest studies and news). Now it's time to turn all this knowledge into practical advice on how to eat every day.

But before we get to meal plans, recipes, and other specifics, we want to introduce you to the foundation of the Smart Fat Solution, because that is the framework that will ultimately help you "smart-fat" all your food for life, after Day 30 of the Thirty-Day Plan, without a recipe or a meal plan, no matter where you are or what you're faced with when it's time to eat.

What to Eat Every Day
for the Rest of Your Life: 5-5-10

You don't need to remember how many calories are in a cup of berries or how many grams of sugar are in a teaspoon (four, if you're wondering). All you have to remember are three numbers: 5, 5, and 10:

- Five (5) servings of smart fat every day
- Five (5) servings of clean protein every day
- Ten (10) servings of fiber every day

You don't have to create a "perfect plate" with precisely balanced amounts of fat, protein, and fiber every time you have a meal or snack. Just remember 5-5-10 (servings) as a minimum, not a maximum—a framework or template for your daily diet. What you're aiming for is a daily intake that you can configure based on your needs and wants. Our Thirty-Day Plan and recipes will help you hit the mark every time, but when you're ready to take off the training wheels and smart-fat food on your own, you'll want 5-5-10 to be second nature—and with a little practice, it will be.

Choosing Your Food:
What to Expect with Your 5-5-10 Day

In order to get the most out of the Smart Fat Solution, particularly for weight loss, follow the Thirty-Day Plan in Chapter 6, which is designed to help you eat 5-5-10 every day. You don't *have* to go off the meal plan after Day 30, as we'll explain in Chapter 7; you can stay on it indefinitely, but eventually you'll want to put together your own meals and snacks as you move toward smart-fatting all your food, for life.

The lists below will give you an idea of what your breakfast, lunch, dinner, and snacks can look like. You don't need to remember percentages, count calories, memorize grams of carbs, or anything else. *Just think 5-5-10.*

SMART MOVE: LEARN TO DO SOME NUMBERS (EVEN THOUGH WE'VE DONE THEM FOR YOU)

We don't want you to get out a calculator every time you feel hungry, but no doubt you've noticed our references throughout this book to "the right amount" or "not enough" of certain foods, and you're probably wondering what those amounts are, exactly. We're going to answer that with specific amounts in the charts and lists to come, and we'll steer you to other sources with that info (and you'll probably get good at reading nutrition labels!).

Don't balk when you see "grams" and "ounces" in the information we're about to provide. It's part of our strategy to help you get some basics down with regard to serving sizes and quantities. Here's the reason: If you understand the numbers behind the food you eat, you'll definitely be more successful at reaching your goals, especially for weight loss.

Grams (g) are the standard unit of measurement on most nutrition labels (for example: "fat: 4g, carbohydrate: 22g, protein: 10g"). *Ounces* are the standard unit of measurement for individual serving sizes of many foods, particularly meats, poultry, fish, nuts, dairy, and beverages. In our 5-5-10 lists, we give many (though not all) individual serving sizes in ounces, followed by gram amounts of fat, protein, and fiber per serving.

We provide this detail in grams and ounces because we want you to get a handle on what's in your food, and we want to share some tips that will simplify your approach to diet and nutrition. For instance, here's a good one: There are about 7 grams of protein in each ounce of an animal protein food. For example, 4 ounces of fish provides approximately 28 grams of pure protein.

Smart Fats: Pick Five (5) a Day

Have *at least* five servings of smart fat a day. You can configure them in your diet as you wish. For instance, you can have one or two per meal, and if you snack twice a day, one per snack; or work a few smart fats into each meal and don't include them in all your snacks. However you choose to do it, *have a minimum of five servings of smart fat daily, and a maximum of ten servings of total fat per day.* If you are trying to lose weight, however, we recommend no more than seven servings of smart or neutral fat per day. This will help keep calorie intake at a level consistent with weight loss.

Unlike protein and fiber, as you'll see, there is no gram amount of smart fat that you'll be aiming for, though we include the fat gram counts below for reference. Think of smart fat intake in terms of servings rather than grams.

- Half an avocado (14 grams)
- 1 ounce (handful) of nuts—our favorites are almonds (14 grams), pistachios (13 grams), pecans (20 grams), walnuts (18 grams), hazelnuts (17 grams), and macadamia nuts (15 grams)
- 1 tablespoon nut oil (from any of the nuts listed above) (approximately 14 grams)[†]
- 1 tablespoon virgin or extra-virgin olive oil (14 grams)
- 1 tablespoon coconut oil (14 grams)
- 1 tablespoon MCT oil (14 grams)
- Two large whole eggs (organic, cage-free) (10 grams)
- Two extra-large whole eggs (organic, cage-free) (12 grams)
- 6–8 ounces fatty fish, such as wild-caught salmon, sardines, or herring (10 grams)
- 1 ounce dark chocolate (at least 70 percent cocoa) (12 grams)

You can also use other neutral fats in moderation, such as butter from grass-fed cows or even some cold-pressed oils like sesame oil. And you may be consuming some fat from foods like grass-fed beef, cage-free and organic poultry, or natural peanut butter. (You can grind your own peanut butter in some food markets, or find one made with organic peanuts, a bit of salt if desired, and a small amount of peanut oil for a consistent texture and spreadability—but no sugar or other additives. See Chapter 7 for more information on peanut and other nut

---

[†] Besides nut, olive, and coconut oils listed here, refer to our list of "Green Light" oils in Chapter 3. For information on the smoke points of various cooking oils and why they matter, see Chapter 10.

butters.) These foods can all be enjoyed in moderation as part of the Smart Food Solution (one to two servings per day), but as fats, they are neutral; therefore, they *don't* count toward your five daily servings of smart fat under the 5-5-10 regime.

EAT FIVE SERVINGS OF SMART FAT DAILY

COCONUT OIL AND CHOLESTEROL

Coconut oil will most likely affect your cholesterol levels. It may raise your total and LDL cholesterol numbers, but it's important to realize that most of this change is positive. Coconut oil will raise good HDL cholesterol levels as well as shift the distribution of your LDL particles so that you have more LDLa (harmless, fluffy) particles and fewer LDLb (small, dense, and harmful) particles, which cause arterial damage. The overall effect on your total cholesterol profile is probably more positive than negative. But if you are taking a statin drug for high cholesterol, or if you have heart disease, it's important to discuss coconut oil intake with your doctor because it *will very likely* raise your numbers and, as a result, may cause your physician to increase your medication dosage. Don't be surprised if your doctor suggests that you choose virgin olive oil, other nut oils, or avocado oil instead of coconut oil.

In addition to the cholesterol issue, saturated fats do increase arterial inflammation and, in one study at least, adversely affect function (albeit in a modest way). Coconut oil is of course a saturated fat. In light of these concerns, Steven asks the patients at his clinic who are at high risk for heart disease to use the other smart fats instead of coconut oil with their eating plans.

For the average healthy person, however, we both believe that coconut oil is a healthy smart fat choice. It's a great fuel for exercise, and it has some clear benefits for your brain and immune system. That's why we've put it firmly in the smart fat category.

Clean Protein: Pick Five (5) a Day

Depending on your age, gender, weight, and weight-loss goals, your protein "number" (number of grams per day) will vary, but we can say without a doubt that most people simply don't get enough protein, in part because of various official recommendations. For instance, the Food and Nutrition Board at the Institute of Medicine recommends daily allowances ranging from 13 grams a day (for a child one to three years old) to 56 grams a day (for adult men); but in our opinion, that's way too little. While the recommended numbers provided by government agencies and medical groups may in fact be the minimum numbers *for basic survival,* they are very far from the desired numbers for optimal health. In fact, we believe they are inadequate when it comes to weight loss. We think the ideal range of protein intake for most adults should be somewhere between 80 and 120 grams. If you're petite, your needs will be closer to 80 grams, but if you're physically large or very active, you'll more likely lean to the higher end of the recommended amount. Please remember that we're talking about *clean* (or *lean,* if you can't find clean) protein sources, not the *mean* protein you find in fried chicken, burgers, sausage, and deli meats. Much has been written about Americans eating too much protein, and no doubt many eat too much mean protein. But because the "official" protein recommendations are so low to begin with, we doubt that most Americans are eating too much.

Aim for a minimum of 20 grams of protein at every meal. If you pick five protein servings a day from foods on our list, you'll easily meet this goal; but we want to point out that 20 grams is a minimum *per meal,* so if you're having a salad for lunch, for instance, keep that in mind. A fiber-rich salad with spinach and other greens, tomatoes, carrots, broccoli, bell peppers, and mushrooms may seem superhealthy, but it's protein-poor. Once in a while a big salad for a meal is fine, but as a general rule, you're better off adding a couple of hardboiled eggs (18 grams) and half a cup of chickpeas (6–7 grams) and making it a smart fat lunch. You'll be getting 24 grams of hunger-curbing protein *and* you'll be satisfied until dinner. Or add one egg, one slice of organic dark-meat turkey bacon (6 grams), and the chickpeas. Once you understand just a few basic numbers, punching up the protein is simple.

If you're trying to lose weight, *we recommend 20 to 30 grams of protein at breakfast.* Protein is *essential* for muscle development—and the muscle cells are fat-burners. Therefore, the more muscle you have, the more effectively you can burn body fat. Eating more protein at breakfast stimulates your metabolism to burn more calories all day, even if you're sitting during much of your workday.

Here are some single-serving protein options that deliver slightly varying amounts of protein. As we've pointed out, roughly 1 ounce of an animal protein food like chicken will deliver 7 grams of protein. That's why so many 4-ounce servings deliver 28 grams of protein! Beef and pork, as you'll see, contain more protein per grams than poultry, and the white meat of chicken contains more than the dark meat.

If you eat five servings of *clean* protein a day, using the list below as a guide, you'll easily fall into the 80–120+ gram range without doing any further calculation, and that's exactly where we want you to be.

- 4 ounces grass-fed beef (about 28 grams) (sirloin has 30 grams; prime rib has 27 grams)
- 4 ounces pastured pork tenderloin (24 grams)
- 4 ounces leg of lamb (33 grams)
- 4 ounces free-range poultry, dark meat (19 grams)
- 4 ounces free-range poultry, breast meat (24 grams)
- 4 ounces coho (silver) salmon (preferably wild-caught) (28 grams)
- 4 ounces tilapia (28 grams)
- Three cage-free, organic eggs (18–24 grams) (large eggs have about 6 grams; jumbo eggs have about 8 grams)
- 1 heaping cup cooked lentils (20 grams)
- 1⅓ cups cooked black beans (20 grams)

- 1⅓ cups shelled edamame (20 grams)
- Two scoops (or one serving, per manufacturer's guidelines) of whey protein powder (20–30 grams)
- Two scoops (or one serving, per manufacturer's guidelines) soy protein powder (20–30 grams)
- Two scoops (or one serving, per manufacturer's guidelines) pea-rice protein powder (20–30 grams)
- 1 cup organic Greek-style yogurt, plain (22 grams) (Greek-style yogurts are generally higher in protein than regular [plain] varieties)
- 1 cup cubed tofu (20 grams)

You may find on this list a lot of animal protein that you aren't used to eating or preparing. But we're not telling you to consume *meat, poultry, and fish* five times a day—though you certainly could, provided, of course, that it was clean. What we *are* telling you is to eat five servings of *protein* a day *from any source*—not just animal foods. In fact, both of us follow this program, and Steven doesn't eat meat at all and Jonny eats it frequently.

As you can see, there are many sources of nonanimal protein. Even a vegetarian can achieve our recommended protein intake. For example, have a protein-rich Smart Fat Shake for breakfast (25 grams of protein), a bowl of black bean soup for lunch (20 grams), edamame and fruit for an afternoon snack (another 10–15 grams), lentil and vegetable Indian curry for dinner (20+ grams), and a bowl of organic Greek-style yogurt with fruit for dessert (21 grams). Voilà! Five servings of clean protein without having to eat meat, fish, or poultry—and this day didn't even include eggs.

Keep in mind that a 4-ounce portion of chicken is actually very modest and will rarely satiate a hungry eater. Six ounces is a more adequate and realistic portion, so 6 ounces of chicken counts as 1.5 servings. Many of our recipes feature servings of clean protein that are between 5 and 8 ounces. Restaurant servings of meat, fish, and poultry are frequently 8 ounces or more—a double serving. (Note: If you eat out regularly, it's especially worth familiarizing yourself with portion sizes and what they look like; restaurant portions are usually too *big*.) In the case of the 8-ounce grass-fed steak, or the 8-ounce serving of chicken or seafood per person in a recipe, figure those amounts as two servings.

As you can see from the examples of 4+ ounces of meat, poultry, and fish, you don't need to consume animal protein five times a day to get to five servings a day.

You can also power up your protein intake significantly by using protein powder, which is why it's such an important ingredient in our morning Smart Fat Shake (see Chapter 10 for recipes). Adding beans and legumes to your meals, as well as plain Greek-style yogurt, is also a smart way to increase your protein intake. See our website, www .SmartFat.com, for more protein sources.

EAT FIVE SERVINGS OF PROTEIN:
At least 20 grams per meal, 80-120 grams per day.

SMART MOVE: EAT MORE PROTEIN, LOSE MORE WEIGHT

We think that most people aren't consuming nearly enough clean protein and that the standard recommendations are too conservative. The Centers for Disease Control and Prevention, for example, recommends 0.8 grams of protein per every kilogram of body weight. (To calculate: Divide your body weight in pounds by 2.2 to convert it to kilograms, then multiply by 0.8.) This works out to about 47 grams of protein for a 128-pound woman—practically half of what we're recommending.

Furthermore, the recommendations don't take into account such questions as whether our hypothetical woman is overweight or under-

CONTINUED ON NEXT PAGE

CONTINUED FROM PAGE 105

weight. Is she pregnant? Is she an athlete? Is she menopausal? How old is she? All of these factors affect her protein intake, but except for basic human survival, 47 grams wouldn't be adequate in any scenario.

Nutritionist Donald Layman has done a significant amount of research on protein and weight loss, and he suggests that if your goal is weight loss—meaning *reducing your level of body fat,* not just lowering your body mass index and the number on your bathroom scale—the ideal amount of protein for you to eat is closer to 1.4 to 1.5 grams per kilogram of body weight—almost twice the amount recommended by some health organizations. (By Layman's formula, our 128-pound woman should be consuming closer to 90 grams of protein, assuming she wants to shed weight, which works out to about double the minimum requirement.)

If you are trying to lose weight and lower your body fat, start by calculating your protein needs using the formula above (convert your weight to kilograms and then multiply by 1.4-1.5), and eat 20-30 grams of protein at breakfast. (For more information on the importance of protein in the morning, see the section on shakes and protein powders later in this chapter. And for more on the importance of losing body fat, not just losing weight, and for tips on the best ways to track your weight loss, see Chapter 7.)

Many popular weight-loss diets recommend protein intake based on a percentage of calories (for instance, the recommendation that 30 percent of your calories should be from protein, or for some diets, a mere 10 percent). But that's a complicated way to think about your daily diet. It's also misleading. Your body needs a certain *amount* of protein, not a certain *percentage* of protein. If a tiny woman who weighs 100 pounds and consumes 1,200 calories a day ate 10 percent of her calories from protein, she'd consume only 30 grams a day. But you don't have to worry about these percentages with the Smart Fat Solution. Just eat five servings of protein every day, and you'll be fine!

Fiber: Pick Ten (10) a Day

Fiber should come from vegetables, fruits, beans, nuts, seeds, a small portion of whole (unprocessed) grains, and perhaps a fiber supplement. Colorful fiber choices will add texture and variety to your plate and help you feel full and satisfied.

Aim for at least 30 grams of fiber every day. To simplify your choices and offer a range of foods, we give you a selection of 3- and 6-gram options in the lists below. Even though we say "pick ten," you could pick five 6-gram servings to get to 30 grams, or you could mix and match some 3- and 6-gram options. How you get there is your choice, depending on your tastes. Just remember where you want to end up!

Vegetables

On average most vegetables have 3 grams of fiber per cup, so 2 cups of vegetables (for a total of 6 grams or more) count as two of your ten servings.

- 1 cup broccoli (2.9 grams)
- 1 cup asparagus (3 grams)
- 1 cup cooked (or 7.5 cups raw) spinach (1 gram)
- 1 cup cooked kale (2.8 grams)
- 1 cup green peas (4 grams)
- 1 cup green beans (2.5 grams)
- Half of a Hass, or California, avocado (5.9 grams)
- One-quarter of the larger, smooth-skinned Florida avocado (4.3 grams)
- Half of a large cooked artichoke (3.3 grams)
- One medium sweet potato (3.5 grams)
- 1 cup boiled purple potatoes (3 grams)
- 1 cup okra (5.2 grams)
- 1 cup chopped tomatoes (1.8 grams)
- 1 cup butternut squash (2.9 grams)

- 1 cup fennel (2.7 grams)
- 1 cup Brussels sprouts (3.3 grams)

Beans and Legumes

On average, 1 cup of cooked beans provides 15 grams of fiber, or five fiber servings. One-half cup of cooked legumes (7–8 grams) counts as 2.5 of your ten fiber servings. Here are ½-cup examples:

- Black or red beans (7.5 grams)
- Lentils (8 grams)
- Chickpeas (7 grams)
- Split peas (8 grams)
- Edamame (7.5 grams)

Fruit

An average cup of fruit has 3 grams of fiber, or one fiber serving.

- One medium apple (3 grams)
- One medium pear (5 grams)
- 1 cup blueberries (3.5 grams)
- One medium orange (3.1 grams)
- ⅓ cup raspberries (2.9 grams)
- 1 cup halved strawberries (3 grams)
- 1 cup sliced peaches (2.8 grams)
- 1½ cups cubed pineapple (3.3 grams)

Select Grains

An average 1-cup serving of grain has 3 grams of fiber, or one fiber serving. Note: Don't have more than one serving of grain at any single meal; limit your grain intake to three servings a day. Less is even better because of the food intolerance challenges that grains can present for many people. We feel it's much better to get your fiber from vegetables, fruits, beans, nuts, and legumes.

- 1 cup steel-cut oats, cooked (equivalent to ¼ cup uncooked) (4 grams)
- ½ cup quinoa, cooked (5 grams) (counts as two servings)
- ½ cup brown rice, cooked (2.6 grams)
- ½ cup wild rice, cooked (3 grams)

Additional Fiber Sources

We include fiber supplements here in case you can't, or don't want to, get all of your fiber from food sources. For an added fiber boost, sprinkle supplements on your steel-cut oats or yogurt or in your morning protein smoothie. A Smart Fat shake with blueberries and almond milk (Steven's typical breakfast) has a whopping 15 grams of fiber. Try these fiber supplement options:

- 1 tablespoon Meta supplement (formerly Metamucil) (3 grams)
- 1⅓ tablespoons ground flaxseed (3 grams)
- 1⅓ tablespoons chia seeds (3 grams)
- One scoop Sunfiber supplement (6 grams)
- 2 teaspoons PaleoFiber supplement (made by Designs for Health) (5 grams)
- One scoop Medibulk fiber powder (made by Thorne Research) (8 grams)
- 1 ounce dark chocolate (1.5 grams)
- 2 tablespoons cocoa powder (hot cocoa) (3.6 grams)

The current fiber intake in the United States is approximately 10 to 15 grams per day, which is way too low. Just for reference, our Paleolithic ancestors, who ate a plant-heavy diet, got at least 50 grams per day! We both make an effort to consume at least 40 and up to 50 grams of fiber every day.

Once you know where to find fiber, it's not hard to get your ten servings (or 30 grams) per day. These numbers are averages; the exact amount of fiber depends on the variety of veggie or fruit, for instance. But the list below shows how simple it can be to reach your goal—

without having to rely on whole grains. Think of eating these foods spaced out over the whole day—for instance, some fruit in the morning and some as a snack. Divide the veggies up between lunch and dinner, or as part of a snack. You can also blend veggies into a Smart Fat Shake (see Chapter 10 for recipes) or include them in a breakfast omelet. Beans and legumes are easy to toss into salads and soups. Even dark chocolate has fiber (even though you've probably always considered dark chocolate a smart fat!).

So here's a day's worth of fiber (30 grams):

- Two pieces of fruit (1 cup of berries or cherries count as one fruit) (6 grams)
- Two handfuls of nuts (about 2 ounces) (6 grams)
- 3 cups veggies (10 grams)
- ½ cup beans in a soup, salad, or side dish (7 grams)
- 1 ounce dark chocolate (1 gram)

EAT TEN SERVINGS OF FIBER: At least 30 grams per day.

SMART MOVE: HOW TO HIT YOUR "GRAM" SLAM (HINT: ROUND UP OR DOWN)

We've now given you three key guidelines on smart fat, protein, and fiber; just remember 5-5-10:

1. *Eat at least five servings of smart fat a day*—up to ten servings of smart and neutral fats and no more than seven fat servings if your goal is weight loss (no gram amount).

2. *Eat at least five servings of protein a day*—a minimum of 20 grams of protein *at each meal.* Aim for 80 to 120 grams per day, depending on your goals and body type.

3. *Eat at least ten servings of fiber a day*—a minimum of 30 grams of fiber daily.

But with regard to grams, *don't be concerned if you don't hit the exact gram amount every time.* It's okay to estimate, and in fact, that's a practical approach that reflects what we all do in real life. The chicken portion may have 25 or 28 grams of protein; the "medium" apple may have 3 grams of fiber or 4. (For tips on estimating portion sizes, see Chapter 7.) Such variations won't hurt you. Feel free to round numbers up or down.

If you are mindful of the guidelines we've given you and make an effort to follow them every day, you will notice the beneficial effect on how you look and feel—even if you're under or over by a few grams. We don't expect you do a lot of arithmetic and check nutritional databases every time you eat. Instead, we want you to learn to use basic knowledge and to make wise, healthful choices. Whether you round up or round down, you're going to win this game!

How to Start Your Smart Fat Solution

To get the most out of the Smart Fat Solution, to see and *feel* results you'll love, we're giving you a Thirty-Day Plan broken down into two phases of ten and twenty days. Thirty days is about how long it takes most of us to make everyday changes that will stick for the long term, and it's ample time for your body (and your mind) to reset and embrace a new way of eating and thinking about your food. (If you're already jumping ahead and wondering what happens on Day 31 and beyond, we've got you covered in Chapter 7.)

During both phases, you'll follow the 5-5-10 guidelines. In addition, during the ten-day Phase 1, we ask you to *skip all alcohol* and *not eat certain foods,* such as grains and potatoes, because both negatively affect blood sugar levels. This restriction, however, is only temporary; you'll be able to reintroduce them back into your regular diet during Phase 2 of the Smart Fat Solution. But we want you to start with a blank slate, metabolically speaking, and if you are experiencing *any* level of insulin or leptin resistance (see Chapter 2), you need to avoid foods that trigger inflammation and blood sugar imbalances. When you remove substances that kick off this cycle, and introduce smart fats, protein, and fiber, you'll get a clearer picture of where you are—and where you want to be.

Here's a preview of Phase 1 and Phase 2, which we cover thoroughly in the next chapter.

Phase 1 Preview: The First Ten Days

- 5-5-10: Five smart fat servings, five protein servings, and ten fiber servings every day
- Unlimited vegetables
- Fruits with a low GL (avoid medium-GL choices such as dried fruits, bananas, and papayas during this phase)
- High-protein/low-carb breakfast (minimum of 20–30 grams protein)
- No grains and no flour products, including breakfast cereals, breads, pastas, crackers, and cookies
- No potatoes
- No alcohol
- Hydration: Drink at least four to eight cups of hydrating fluid every day (water, carbonated water, and herbal teas).
  —In addition to water, if you want to lose weight, include four cups of regular and/or decaf green tea daily; green tea contains a compound known as EGCG (epigallocatechin gallate), which helps you lose weight. (See Chapter 8 for more on EGCG.)
  —You may also have one to two cups of coffee daily, but only in addition to water and tea, not as a substitute.
- Start a personalized Smart Supplement plan on Day 1 (see Chapter 8).

Phase 2 Preview: The Next Twenty Days (and Beyond)

- Continue 5-5-10: five smart fat servings, five protein servings, and ten fiber servings every day.
- Continue unlimited vegetables.
- Fruits: If you've hit your desired weight, continue to enjoy low-GL fruits; occasionally, eat medium-GL fruits in moderation. If you haven't achieved your desired weight, continue to avoid medium-GL fruits.
- Breakfast: If you are at your desired weight, aim for 20 grams of protein. For continued weight loss, continue to eat a minimum of 20–30 grams protein.
- Grains and flour products: If you are at your desired weight, you may add moderate amounts of pasta (al dente) or 1-cup portions of medium-GL grains (wild rice, quinoa, steel-cut oats, brown rice), but limit these to one serving per day. Treat bread and white rice like birthday cake—that is, it's okay for a special occasion, but not for everyday eating. For continued weight loss, continue to avoid grains and flour products.
- Potatoes: Instead of high-GL baked russet potatoes, choose medium-GL potatoes, such as sweet potatoes or purple potatoes.
- Alcohol: If you are at your desired weight, one to two servings of alcohol, five days per week. For continued weight loss, one serving three days per week, with a meal. If you can't limit intake to one serving, then continue to avoid alcohol altogether until you reach your goal weight.
- Hydration: Maintain hydration with four to eight cups of fluid per day. For continued weight loss, drink four cups of regular and/or decaffeinated tea daily.
- Continue your personalized Smart Supplement plan (see Chapter 8).

You can stay on Phase 2 for life, not just for twenty days, if you stay within the guidelines above and continue to smart-fat your daily meals using the 5-5-10 principle.

Follow these two phases of the Smart Fat Solution and you'll feel different—*better*—after ten days and even better again after twenty more. Some of you might feel better after only two or three days. It's important (and motivating!) to be mindful of how you react to this new way of eating, so stay attuned to how you're feeling and make some notes, if you'd like. You don't need to keep a food diary if you're adhering to the plan (we'll talk more about food diaries in Chapter 7), but you may want to pay special attention to what is working best for you and what you'd like to tweak once you're off the Thirty-Day Plan. If you're tracking weight loss, see Chapter 7 for our recommendations.

At this point, we realize that you may have some nuts-and-bolts questions, such as:

- What should I always have in my fridge and pantry?
- Can I still have dessert?
- What about alcohol?
- Should I give up gluten?
- How much pasta can I have? Does it have to be whole grain?
- Is it okay to drink cow's milk in my latte?
- Does *everything* need to be organic?
- So, tell me again, can I eat raisins, or not?

We'll get to these questions and more in Chapter 7, where you'll find more practical information and tools to help you stay on track—for life.

So you know about the principle of 5-5-10 servings every day, and you've got a clear sense of what you'll be eating on the Thirty-Day Plan and beyond. You're just about ready to get started, but let's take a moment to look at the first meal of the day, breakfast—probably the biggest change we're asking you to make.

GOOD FOODS THAT WORK OVERTIME

You've probably noticed that some foods fall into more than one of our must-have categories of smart fat, protein, and fiber:

- Nuts and seeds: smart fat and fiber
- Beans and legumes: protein and fiber
- Dark chocolate: smart fat and fiber
- Eggs: smart fat and protein
- Fish: smart fat and protein

We love it when great-tasting foods do more than one thing! This is smart double-dipping.

Breakfast: More Important Than Ever

For some of you, eating a Smart Fat breakfast—or *any* breakfast—may represent a huge lifestyle shift, so we want to take a moment and walk you through this important first meal of the day—and of the Smart Fat Solution.

A high-protein/low-carb breakfast, with 20–30 grams of protein, will rev your metabolism and fuel your brain and your body simultaneously. If you kick off your day with a smart fat breakfast, you'll feel terrific whether your breakfast consists of a quick-and-easy morning Smart Fat Shake or you take a little time to prepare a delicious omelet or a bowl of hearty, fiber-rich steel-cut oats mixed with some protein powder. You may be used to a breakfast of cereal, juice, toast, and coffee, or something similar with a high glycemic load. You may not like the idea of cooking first thing in the morning (and you may mistakenly assume that eating eggs for breakfast, or at any meal, will do crazy things to your cholesterol—it won't! See more on eggs in Chapter 7). Or, you may skip the food altogether in the morning and go for just a beverage. But it's time to wake up and smell the coffee, *and eat something smart!*

We're here to help you fix—in both senses of the word—your breakfast.

The Smart Fat Shake: Protein Perfection in a Glass

There are days when you have time to make breakfast and days when you feel rushed. If you're like most of us, you'll more often feel rushed! That's why we've created our Smart Fat Shake, which delivers the right amount of smart fat, protein, and fiber quickly and deliciously. It's easy to prepare in minutes, with a blender and some key ingredients that are easy to keep on hand. Best of all, you can vary the flavors with some simple substitutions. We both start nearly every day of the week with a Smart Fat Shake. Take it from us—it does the trick!

You'll find Smart Fat Shake recipes in Chapter 10, but here are the key ingredients:

- Frozen fruit (berries, cherries, and peaches are great—frozen fruit has the same nutrients as fresh, they're available year-round, they're prewashed and ready to use, they're generally cheaper than fresh, and they deliver the right texture as well as a refreshingly cold temperature)
- Almond milk *(unsweetened)*, coconut milk beverage (in a carton, not a can), organic (non-GMO) soy milk, or organic cow's milk
- A serving of protein powder
- Fiber supplement if necessary (some protein powders contain extra fiber, but if not, add chia seeds, ground flaxseeds, Medibulk (Thorne Research), PaleoFiber (Designs for Health), or Sunfiber supplements)
- A smart fat like almond butter, MCT oil, 1–2 tablespoons of chia seeds or ground flaxseeds, or 1 tablespoon of nut oil, including coconut oil (these won't alter or mask the fruity flavor of your shake)

Put everything in a blender, hit the button, then pour and enjoy! Start to finish, it takes about two minutes to make. Play around with flavors, textures, and different combinations. If you don't want to add a dose of smart fat to your shake, just make sure that you have some on the side, such as almond butter on apple slices or MCT oil in your coffee.

Our Smart Fat Shake offers clean protein, smart fat, fabulous fiber, and fluid—and a superfast solution to feeling satisfied and hydrated. Have the Smart Fat Shake for breakfast or use it as a meal replacement from time to time. Try a shake—or make a mini-version—as a snack, too!

PICK YOUR POWDER: WHEY TO GO!

You may think that protein powder supplements are just for Arnold Schwarzenegger wannabees, but they have been mainstream among the nutrition-savvy for years. Protein powder is a critical ingredient in our Smart Fat Shake, plus it can turn a bowl of regular steel-cut oats into a protein-perfect breakfast food.

You can purchase large canisters (the most cost-effective) or single-serving packets (more expensive, but a good idea if you're on the go or you want to try out different types of powders and aren't ready to "commit" to the big container). And you no longer have to hunt them down in specialty vitamin stores. A well-stocked supermarket, particularly one that has a large selection of organic, natural foods, often has protein powders for sale. You can also find a huge selection online, including our own brand of protein powder, which we formulate especially for our Smart Fat Shake. (Visit www.SmartFat.com for sources.)

There are three main categories of protein powder:

- Whey protein. Whey is derived from cow's milk, so make sure yours comes from grass-fed, hormone-free cows. Yes, it's more expensive, but it's worth it. Bargain shoppers can wind up with a powder that's enriched with pesticides and hormones.

CONTINUED ON NEXT PAGE

CONTINUED FROM PAGE 117

- *Soy protein.* Remember that most of the soy produced in the United States is genetically modified, so only shop for soy protein made from organic, non-GMO soy.
- *Pea protein or brown rice protein.* These vegetarian options are increasingly popular among people who want to avoid both soy and animal products.

If you have no food (dairy) sensitivities or allergies, we think whey protein powder is the way to go. Not only do we prefer its taste and texture (whey makes for a creamier shake), but whey supports your immune system and builds muscle mass better than soy and pea-rice proteins. There's also a fair amount of research showing that whey is helpful for weight loss and reduces several risk factors for Metabolic Syndrome.

That said, if you can't consume dairy, soy is a good option. Soy protein has been shown to help reduce symptoms of menopause and lower the risk of certain cancers.

Pea-rice protein powders (all-pea protein, all–brown rice protein, or more likely a combination) are good choices for people who want to avoid animal protein and soy altogether. Up to 20 percent of people may be soy and/or dairy intolerant, so pea-rice protein powders are an excellent option if you are on an elimination diet for food intolerances.

Manufacturers continue to release protein powders made from alternative sources, such as hemp and sacha inchi, a traditional plant from tropical South America, but we want to steer you to the most proven protein sources available—whey, soy, and pea-rice powders. Experiment with what suits you best.

We've given you the framework of 5-5-10 servings per day, and we've outlined the two phases of the Smart Fat Solution Thirty-Day Plan. In the next chapter you get all the meal plans to take you through thirty life-changing days, so keep reading!

CHAPTER 6

The Thirty-Day Plan
of Smart Fat Meals

Here's your Thirty-Day Plan of menus, divided into the ten-day Phase 1 (Days 1–10) and the twenty-day Phase 2 (Days 11–30) that we introduced in Chapter 5. You'll find many of the recipes in Chapter 10 (and more on our website at www.SmartFat.com). We've indicated the dishes below that have a recipe either in the book (*) or on our website (**).

You may be wondering whether you have to cook the recipes and follow the daily meal plans *exactly* as presented in order to lose weight and reap the health benefits of the Smart Fat Solution. The short answer is, no. But here's the thing: The meal plans and recipes are carefully calibrated to give you the *just-right amounts* of smart fat, protein, and fiber for success—whatever your dietary and health goals may be. That's why we urge you to follow the Thirty-Day Plan as closely as you can for the thirty days. The first ten days are especially important as your body gets used to smart fat eating and you start to break free from dangerous insulin and leptin resistance.

If you don't want to use the recipes, that's okay. You may wish to use your own recipes or change the flavors to suit your taste buds. (For some meals, we've suggested general ideas for main dishes and sides—like a grilled sirloin steak or a baked sweet potato—but we don't include a recipe under the assumption that you'll prepare these basic foods as you wish.) It's fine if you choose to use this Thirty-Day Plan as an inspiration for your own breakfasts, lunches, and dinners—but it's absolutely essential to follow the 5-5-10 guidelines for both phases, even when you're adapting your own recipes. For instance, if you have a recipe for turkey chili that you like better than ours, go for it! Just make sure that the ingredients you use are in line with the phases as outlined. (That's so important that we're repeating those guidelines in boxes for quick reference.) It's pretty simple to cook using your own recipes, if you think of it that way.

We also offer a daily snack suggestion in our meal plan, which you are free to have at any time of the day when you feel you need it most. We think a snack between lunch and dinner is the best time, but it depends on your schedule. You may have a really long stretch between breakfast and lunch some days, so that's when you'll probably want a little something extra. It's up to you—but we do suggest you avoid eating right before bed, as well as midnight trips to the refrigerator, unless you are trying to gain weight. Sumo wrestlers, who do just that, have taught us that eating before bedtime most definitely promotes weight gain!

One more note: The Thirty-Day Plan is presented as Days 1 through 30. You're free to kick off this plan any day of the week, but in our experience, starting on Sunday works well for many people's schedules. We encourage you to prepare a soup of the week on weekends, or whenever you have some free time. We also reserve some "goodies" for weekend meals (if you start this on a Sunday, those meals fall on the weekends, like the brunch idea on Day 21), and include some recipes that are more suitable for a weekend night.

Welcome to Phase 1—you're going to feel great!

Phase 1:
The First Ten Days, Day 1 Through Day 10

Phase 1 at a Glance

- 5-5-10: Five smart fat servings, five protein servings, and ten fiber servings every day
- Unlimited vegetables
- Fruits with a low GL (avoid medium-GL choices such as dried fruits, bananas, and papayas during this phase)
- High-protein/low-carb breakfast (minimum of 20–30 grams protein)
- No grains and no flour products, including breakfast cereals, breads, pastas, crackers, and cookies
- No potatoes
- No alcohol
- Hydration: Drink at least four to eight cups of hydrating fluid every day (water, carbonated water, and herbal teas).
  —In addition to water, if you want to lose weight, include four cups of regular and/or decaf green tea daily; green tea contains a compound known as EGCG (epigallocatechin gallate), which helps you lose weight. (See Chapter 8 for more on EGCG.)
  —You may also have one to two cups of coffee daily, but only in addition to water and tea, not as a substitute.
- Start a personalized Smart Supplement plan on Day 1 (see Chapter 8).

DAY 1

Breakfast

Omelet with Sweet Onion, Red Bell Pepper, and Kale*

Tea, Coffee, or Hot Unsweetened Cocoa

Lunch

    Grilled Lamb Chops*

    Tossed Smart Green Salad with Vinaigrette Dressing

    Unsweetened Ice Tea

Snack

    Ratatouille with Cannellini Beans (soup/lunch of the week)**

Dinner

    Sautéed Turkey Loins with Italian Herbs*

    Swiss Chard, Grated Beets, and Garlic

    Organic Hard Cheese of Choice and Fruit

DAY 2

Breakfast

    Smart Fat Shake: Vanilla, Blueberry, and Spinach*

    Tea, Coffee, or Hot Unsweetened Cocoa

Lunch

    Grilled Free-Range Chicken Salad with Vinaigrette Dressing

    Unsweetened Iced Tea

Snack

    Dark Chocolate and Almonds (1 ounce of each)

    Protein Bar

Dinner

    Spinach and Mushroom Frittata*

    Tomato, Cucumber, and Kalamata Olive Salad

DAY 3

Breakfast

    Greek Yogurt (plain, organic) with Berries and Mixed Nuts

    Tea, Coffee, or Hot Unsweetened Cocoa

Lunch

    Shrimp, Fennel, and Cannellini Bean Salad with

        Orange Vinaigrette Dressing

    Unsweetened Iced Tea

Snack

    Guacamole with Jicama and Red Bell Pepper

    Smart Fat Shake of Your Choice

Dinner

    Sirloin Steak Chili

    Fruit and Cheese

DAY 4

Breakfast

    Smart Fat Shake: Chocolate, Cherry and Spinach*

    Tea, Coffee, or Hot Unsweetened Cocoa

Lunch

    Ratatouille with Cannellini Beans

    Apple

Snack

    Dark Chocolate and Macadamia Nuts (1 ounce of each)

    Protein Bar

Dinner

    Roasted Chicken with Mediterranean Herbs*

    Sliced Pear with Gorgonzola and Walnuts

DAY 5

Breakfast

    Eggs Fried in Olive Oil with Garlic and Sautéed Kale

    Tea, Coffee, or Hot Unsweetened Cocoa

Lunch

    Ratatouille with Cannellini Beans

    Unsweetened Ice Tea

Snack

    Smart Fat Shake of Your Choice

Dinner

    Sautéed Chicken with Fennel and Zucchini Slices

    Arugula Salad with Toasted Pine Nuts and Lemony Vinaigrette

DAY 6

Breakfast
 Smart Fat Shake: Vanilla-Peach Chia Seed
 Tea, Coffee, or Hot Unsweetened Cocoa
Lunch
 Shrimp and Veggie Kebobs
 Unsweetened Iced Tea
Snack
 Dark Chocolate and Almonds (1 ounce of each)
Dinner
 Grilled Bronzino (European sea bass) with Lemon Zest,
  Mediterranean Herbs, and Virgin Olive Oil
 White Bean Salad*
 Quick Kale Sauté

DAY 7

Breakfast
 Smoked Salmon, Green Onion, Egg Scramble
 Tea, Coffee, or Hot Unsweetened Cocoa
Lunch
 Turkey Chili**
 Unsweetened Iced Tea
Snack
 Smoked Oysters with Avocado on Cucumber Slices*
Dinner
 Turkey Meatballs with Butternut Squash and Mixed Vegetables*
 Avocado, Cucumber, and Garbanzo Salad*

DAY 8

Breakfast
 Western Omelet, Fruit Salad with Greek Yogurt
 Tea, Coffee, or Hot Unsweetened Cocoa

Lunch

    Butternut Squash Soup with Ginger and Fennel*

    Sliced Turkey and Avocado and Lettuce Wrap

    Strawberries

Snack

    Guacamole with Jicama and Red Bell Pepper*

Dinner

    Roasted Grass-Fed Bison and Root Vegetables*

DAY 9

Breakfast

    Smart Fat Shake: Chocolate-Berry Chia Seed

    Tea, Coffee, or Hot Unsweetened Cocoa

Lunch

    Crab Cakes with Quinoa, Mango Salsa, Green Salad*

    Unsweetened Iced Tea

Snack

    Apple with Dark Chocolate Drizzle*

Dinner

    Marinated Flank Steak over Mixed Green Salad*

DAY 10

Breakfast

    Smart Fat Shake: Vanilla, Cherry, and Kale*

    Tea, Coffee, or Hot Unsweetened Cocoa

Lunch

    Turkey Chili

    Orange

Snack

    Apple and Almonds

Dinner

    Chicken with Pecan-Herb Crust*

    Roasted Beets and Butternut Squash**

Phase 2:
Twenty More Days—Day 11 Through Day 30

Congrats! You made it! Ten days and you're feeling great, right? Time to move to Phase 2 meal plans (the phase guidelines from the last chapter are repeated below). You can start to add a few things back into your diet, most notably alcohol and low-GL grains. If you think you feel good after ten days, just wait until you see how you feel after another twenty. You're going to want to eat this way for life.

Phase 2 at a Glance

- Continue 5-5-10: five smart fat servings, five protein servings, and ten fiber servings every day.
- Continue unlimited vegetables.
- Fruits: If you've hit your desired weight, continue to enjoy low-GL fruits; occasionally, eat medium-GL fruits in moderation. If you haven't achieved your desired weight, continue to avoid medium-GL fruits.
- Breakfast: If you are at your desired weight, aim for 20 grams of protein. For continued weight loss, continue to eat a minimum of 20–30 grams protein.
- Grains and flour products: If you are at your desired weight, you may add moderate amounts of pasta (al dente) or 1-cup portions of medium-GL grains (wild rice, quinoa, steel-cut oats, brown rice), but limit these to one serving per day. Treat bread and white rice like birthday cake—that is, it's okay for a special occasion, but not for everyday eating. For continued weight loss, continue to avoid grains and flour products.
- Potatoes: Instead of high-GL baked russet potatoes, choose medium-GL potatoes, such as sweet potatoes or purple potatoes.
- Alcohol: If you are at your desired weight, one to two servings of alcohol, five days per week. For continued weight loss, one serv-

ing three days per week, with a meal. If you can't limit intake to one serving, then continue to avoid alcohol altogether until you reach your goal weight.

- Hydration: Maintain hydration with four to eight cups of fluid per day. For continued weight loss, drink four cups of regular and/or decaffeinated tea daily.

- Continue your personalized Smart Supplement plan (see Chapter 8).

DAY 11

Breakfast
Smart Fat Shake: Chocolate and Strawberry*
Tea, Coffee, or Hot Unsweetened Cocoa
Lunch
Grilled Chicken, Spinach, and Strawberry Salad
Snack
Mixed Nuts and Berries
Dinner
Crab Cakes with Quinoa*
Roasted Asparagus, Red Onion, and Orange Vinaigrette

DAY 12

Breakfast
Scrambled Eggs with Veggies and Ham
Tea, Coffee, or Hot Unsweetened Cocoa
Lunch
Grass-Fed Burgers with Sweet Potato Fries
Unsweetened Ice Tea
Snack
Hardboiled Egg and Sliced Avocado
Dinner
Middle Eastern Chicken Sauté*
Wild Rice and Quinoa with Kale and Slivered Almonds*

DAY 13

Breakfast
    Smart Fat Shake: Vanilla-Peach Chia Seed
    Tea, Coffee, or Hot Unsweetened Cocoa
Lunch
    Apple-Walnut Chicken Salad
Snack
    Sliced Pear with Dark Chocolate Swirl and Pecans*
Dinner
    Baked White Fish with Orange Marinade*
    Bok Choy and Shiitake Mushrooms with Brown Rice

DAY 14

Breakfast
    Steel-Cut Oatmeal with Vanilla Protein Powder, Berries, and
        Sliced Almonds**
    Tea, Coffee, or Hot Unsweetened Cocoa
Lunch
    Roasted Chicken Breasts with Arugula and Fennel Salad
Snack
    Smart Fat Shake of Your Choice
Dinner
    Wild Mushroom Soufflé*
    Smart Mixed Green Salad with Italian Dressing

DAY 15

Breakfast
    Smart Fat Shake: Vanilla, Blueberry, and Spinach
    Tea, Coffee, or Hot Unsweetened Cocoa
Lunch
    Wild Rice and Quinoa with Kale and Slivered Almonds*
    Unsweetened Iced Tea

Snack

  Smoked Salmon with Sliced Cucumbers

Dinner

  Baked Halibut with Almond Crust

  Swiss Chard with Garlic Sautéed in Coconut Oil

  Purple Potatoes with Garlic, Herbs, and Parsley*

  Sliced Fruit

DAY 16

Breakfast

  Smart Fat Shake: Chocolate, Cherry, and Spinach*

  Tea, Coffee, or Hot Unsweetened Cocoa

Lunch

  Wild Rice and Quinoa with Kale and Slivered Almonds*

Snack

  Guacamole with Sliced Carrot and Celery

Dinner

  Broiled Oysters with Walnut, Parmesan Cheese, and Parsley Crust*

  Spinach and Kale Salad with Walnuts

  Fruit Salad with Mint, Lemon Rind, and Greek Yogurt

DAY 17

Breakfast

  Steel-Cut Oatmeal with Vanilla Protein Powder, Berries, and
    Sliced Almonds**

  Tea, Coffee, or Hot Unsweetened Cocoa

Lunch

  Smart Mixed Green Salad with Crab and Orange Vinaigrette
    Dressing

  Unsweetened Iced Tea

Snack

  Dark Chocolate and Pistachios (1 ounce of each)

Dinner

Broiled (or Grilled) Scallops with Shredded Beet and Orange Rind**

Green Beans Cooked with Organic Bacon

Fresh Strawberries with Nuts and Organic Greek Yogurt

DAY 18

Breakfast

Scrambled Eggs with Salsa and a Side of Black Beans

Tea, Coffee, or Hot Unsweetened Cocoa

Lunch

Sautéed Turkey Loin with Smart Green Salad

Unsweetened Ice Tea

Snack

Dark Chocolate and Almonds (1 ounce of each)

Dinner

Beef Stew*

Romaine Lettuce Salad with Avocado and Sesame Seeds

DAY 19

Breakfast

Smart Fat Shake of Your Choice

Tea, Coffee, or Hot Unsweetened Cocoa

Lunch

Minestrone Soup**

Orange

Snack

Pistachios

Protein Bar

Dinner

Avocado, Tomato, and Fresh Mozzarella Salad with Mint

Moroccan Chicken Stew*

Raspberries with Organic, Fresh Whipped Cream

DAY 20

Breakfast

Smart Fat Shake of Your Choice

Tea, Coffee, or Hot Unsweetened Cocoa

Lunch

Turkey Chili

Snack

Organic Greek Yogurt and Apple

Dinner

Grilled Sirloin Steak

Sautéed Swiss Chard with Garlic and Italian Herbs*

Wild Rice and Quinoa with Kale and Slivered Almonds

DAY 21

Brunch

Frittata with Kale, Tomato, and Bacon (organic pork, turkey, or
veggie bacon)

Tea, Coffee, or Hot Unsweetened Cocoa

Snack

Crab Avocado Dip*

Dinner

Roasted Chicken with Mediterranean Herbs*

Roasted Beets

Sautéed Kale with Garlic and Lemon*

DAY 22

Breakfast

Spinach Quiche with Sweet Potato Fries

Tea, Coffee, or Hot Unsweetened Cocoa

Lunch

Gumbo**

Orange

Snack

   Nut Butter with Celery Sticks and/or Sliced Apple

Dinner

   Tandoori Chicken*

   Vegetable Korma*

   Raita (Cucumber and Yogurt Salad)*

   Sliced Mango

DAY 23

Breakfast

   Smart Fat Shake: Vanilla, Blueberry, and Spinach

   Tea, Coffee, or Hot Unsweetened Cocoa

Lunch

   Tandoori Chicken and Korma Leftovers

   Pear

Snack

   Dark Chocolate and Pecans (1 ounce of each)

Dinner

   Smart Lemon-Butter Sauce with Salmon and Brussels Sprouts*

   Black Beans

DAY 24

Breakfast

   Smart Fat Shake: Chocolate, Cherry, and Spinach*

   Tea, Coffee, or Hot Unsweetened Cocoa

Lunch

   Gumbo**

Snack

   Dark Chocolate and Almonds (1 ounce of each)

Dinner

   Chicken Satay Skewers with Cabbage Wraps and Almond
      Butter–Coconut Milk Sauce*

   Hard Cheese and Sliced Pear

DAY 25

Breakfast

Steel-Cut Oatmeal with Vanilla Protein Powder, Nuts, and Apple**

Tea, Coffee, or Hot Unsweetened Cocoa

Lunch

Veggie Chili

Snack

Smart Fat Shake of Your Choice

Dinner

Grilled Salmon with Lemon, Dill, Chili, and Paprika

Quinoa with Kale, Mushrooms, and Onions

Dark Chocolate

DAY 26

Breakfast

Smart Fat Shake: Vanilla-Peach Chia Seed

Tea, Coffee, or Hot Unsweetened Cocoa

Lunch

Gumbo**

Snack

Pistachios and Tangerine

Dinner

Pork Tenderloin with Mediterranean Herbs**

Sautéed Swiss Chard with Garlic

Baked Sweet Potato

DAY 27

Breakfast

Smart Fat Shake: Chocolate-Berry Chia Seed

Tea, Coffee, or Hot Unsweetened Cocoa

Lunch

Lentil Curry*

Snack
    Macadamia Nuts and Dark Chocolate (1 ounce of each)
Dinner
    Steak Kebobs with Pineapple, Onion, and Bell Pepper*

DAY 28

Breakfast
    Huevos Rancheros (Fried Eggs with Black Beans and Salsa)
    Tea, Coffee, or Hot Unsweetened Cocoa
Lunch
    Mushroom-Nut Pâté*
    Roasted Brussels Sprouts with Chopped Walnuts
Snack
    Asian Pear, Gorgonzola Cheese, Walnuts, and Raspberries*
Dinner
    Coconut Milk Curry with Shrimp and Broccoli*
    Dark Chocolate

DAY 29

Breakfast
    Smart Fat Shake: Vanilla, Cherry, and Kale*
    Tea, Coffee, or Hot Unsweetened Cocoa
Lunch
    Grilled Chicken Salad with Italian Dressing
    Iced Tea
Snack
    Hard-boiled Egg
Dinner
    Sautéed Salmon
    Steamed Broccoli with Smart Lemon Butter Sauce*
    Wild Rice
    Dark Chocolate

DAY 30

Breakfast
  Vegetable Omelet
  Tea, Coffee, or Hot Unsweetened Cocoa

Lunch
  Minestrone Soup
  Iced Tea

Snack
  Macadamia Nuts and Apple

Dinner
  Grilled Grass-fed Tenderloin Steak
  Sautéed Green Beans with Garlic
  Mashed Roasted Cauliflower

So we come to the end of our suggested menus for the Thirty-Day Plan of the Smart Fat Solution. As we've said, you'll find many of the recipes in Chapter 10 and at www.SmartFat.com, but now, let's turn to some of those nuts-and-bolts questions you may have had to this point.

CHAPTER 7

The Smart Fat User's Guide

OUR THIRTY-DAY PLAN AND RECIPES (see Chapter 10) take the guesswork out of what to eat, but eventually it will be Day 31.

Now what? Well, that depends on your goals.

Maybe you've been losing weight over the course of the first thirty days, but you're still not where you want to be. You feel like you have a bit (or even more than a bit) to go. If that's your situation, please review both phases of the Thirty-Day Plan and continue to follow the modifications in Phase 2 for continued weight loss. With a little persistence, and a touch of patience, you'll definitely get to a weight you can feel good about.

Then there will be those of you who are pretty satisfied at the end of the first thirty days! You lost some weight, and you feel fantastic—so healthy and so strong that you want to continue your Smart Fat Solution for the rest of your life. And why wouldn't you? You've finally found a delicious, simple way of eating that works, and you've made a commitment to smart-fat all your food.

Of course you can continue to use the recipes and modify the flavors or make smart fat substitutions that work for you. But let's be real. You're not going to carry around this book everywhere you go for the rest of your life. At some point—whether you're in the grocery store, sitting in a restaurant, or standing in front of the refrigerator trying to figure out what to make for dinner—you are going to ask the hard questions about what to eat. We want to answer them, preferably before you put that food in your shopping cart, place your order, or open the fridge.

Because your questions may have to do with what choices to make throughout the course of your day, we'll start with breakfast, head for lunch and some smart snacking, and end with dinner—with a couple of side trips in between, including tips on what to do if you hit the dreaded "plateau," whether or not you should keep a food diary (spoiler alert: Yep, they work), and the ultimate answer to that age-old question: "Should I throw away my bathroom scale?" (Short answer: Maybe it's time to get a new scale—we'll tell you why.)

Consider this chapter your Smart Fat User's Guide, for life.

Breakfast Smarts

One reason we recommend our Smart Fat Shake for breakfast is because it's so simple to prepare and it's *so fast,* which is particularly valuable in the morning when you may be rushed and ready to start your day. But even if you're ready to "shake it," you may still have some questions about that first meal of the day.

What's wrong with a glass of orange juice?

Nothing, if you like a bolt of sugar and the resulting havoc it wreaks on your metabolism. In our opinion, and in the opinions of many experts on health and nutrition, orange juice is little more than sugar water, despite its place of honor on the American breakfast table. Even if the primary ingredients are oranges, its high-sugar, high-calorie payload doesn't compare to an actual orange.

An 8-ounce glass of orange juice, for instance, has 23 grams of sugar—that's not *added* sugar, that's just concentrated fruit sugars—

more than 100 calories, and zero grams of fiber. An average whole orange, on the other hand, is a nutrient-packed, low-GL food, with about 4 grams of beneficial fiber to fill you up and loads of vitamin C.

Ditch the juice; eat the fruit.

You can make the same argument for other whole fruits that are frequently turned into juices, such as apples. You get some sugar, sure, but with a whole fruit, you get fiber, water, vitamins, minerals, and disease-fighting phytochemicals like flavonoids—all in a package that is low-glycemic, particularly so when compared with its sugary liquid sister.

Here's the problem with taking in calories from juice—without any protein or fiber. When you drink juice, you consume 100 calories, but you don't feel full, and you will eat the same amount of food whether you had the juice or not. An 8-ounce glass of juice every day for a year adds up an extra 36,500 calories, which will add about 11 pounds of fat to your frame. (It takes 3,500 calories to make 1 pound of fat). We know we said that we weren't going to count calories, but here's a case where the numbers tell the story. In contrast, when you eat an orange, you feel full from the fiber and you benefit from its many nutrients. Say it with us this time: *Ditch the juice; eat the fruit.*

Despite the efforts of Big Food to position fruit juice as a health food, it's anything but. Fruit juice is a habit, a comfort food that we've been putting on the breakfast table for way too long. Even worse, it has fueled today's billion-dollar "juice beverage" industry, which has given us fruit-flavored drinks that are no better than soda—possibly worse, because they are masquerading as healthy choices, and children and young adults are their target audiences. At least soda doesn't pretend. (And don't be seduced by juices that are "enriched" with calcium and vitamin D. If you were eating real fruit instead of a highly sweetened beverage, you wouldn't need it to be "enriched.")

Okay, so what about "juicing"? That's better, isn't it?

Juicing is more popular than ever, with juice bars springing up all over the place. We're also seeing a proliferation of expensive "cold-pressed" juices and companies selling juice-based detox programs. Freshly made vegetable and fruit juices can be a way to obtain some vitamins or minerals from nearly anything in the produce section. And for people who aren't getting many vegetables and fruits in their diet, juicing can be a way for them to get some modest nutritional value.

But there are some negatives to this new health sensation. Yes, you get a nutritionally dense beverage made from fresh and healthy real vegetables and fruit. But what you *don't* get is fiber, which usually gets left behind with the pulp. And that's the big trade-off with juicing—you lose the fiber.

The other negative thing about juicing is that juice is still juice. Which means, given the fact that most drinks are heavy with sweet fruits, you're looking at a potentially high glycemic load. This is not a problem with an all-green juice made from, say, spinach, kale, and cucumber, but more often than not, commercial juice bars will front-load drinks with apples and carrots to make it sweet, which only adds a lot of sugar to the mix.

There's a big distinction between juicing and a popular process called "blending." Juicing is using an extractor to separate the pulp from the juice and then drinking just the latter. Blending is something you do with a high-powered machine like a Vita Mix: You throw the entire fruit or vegetable into the machine, and it liquefies everything. This makes for an incredibly rich, nutrient-dense beverage in which no component of the vegetable or fruit is lost—not the pulp, the fiber, the peel, or even, sometimes, the pit. We're big fans of blenders for just this reason.

Regular juicing is much more hit and miss. One famous chain of national juice bars sells "healthy" fruit juice mixes that seem to us to be ready-made for inducing a diabetic coma. (We're exaggerating, but not by much!) Freshly made apple or orange juice might taste better than what you buy in the store, and even might have a few more nutrients and a few less preservatives, but it's still a big sugar shock for your system. If you do juice, frontload the mix with mostly fresh vegetables, and you should be fine. Or better yet, get yourself a blender!

I'm not used to eating eggs—I can't shake the idea that they'll raise my cholesterol.

The notion that dietary cholesterol, such as the natural cholesterol found in eggs, contributes to causing heart disease was even dismissed by Ancel Keys, who was an early proponent of the theory that cholesterol causes heart disease. Keys fervently believed that cholesterol in the *blood* (and saturated fat in the *diet*) were important causes of heart disease, but even he never thought that the cholesterol we *eat* had much to do with anything. He has been widely quoted as saying, in 1997, "There's no connection whatsoever between the cholesterol in food and cholesterol in the blood. And we've known that all along. Cholesterol in the diet doesn't matter at all."

The funny thing is that only about one-third of the fat in an egg is saturated fat anyway; the majority of it is monounsaturated fat—the same kind of fat found in olive oil. And in any case, even when saturated fat *does* raise total blood cholesterol slightly, it still seems to have an overall beneficial effect, lowering inflammatory LDL particles while raising HDL. Even the conservative Harvard School of Public Health admits that the equivalent of one egg a day (or seven in one week) poses no threat to health—a statement backed up by considerable research.

Our personal belief is that if your eggs are coming from free-range, organically raised chickens (*not* the kind raised in battery cages by big producers and fed a diet of pesticide-tainted grain), you have little to fear from egg yolks and a lot to gain. Besides protein, egg yolks are a wonderful source of the brain nutrient choline, as well as lutein and zeaxanthin, two of the superstars of eye nutrition. But if your eggs are from toxic, factory-farmed chickens, unfortunately you're better off with less-nutrient-dense egg white omelets. (The Smart Fat Solution adage—*if you can't eat clean, eat lean*—goes for eggs too.)

You might encounter conventional supermarket eggs that make claims about their hens being fed a diet "enriched" with omega-3s, but remember: Such animals might still eat a nonorganic diet of pesticide-sprayed chickenfeed, so ensure the eggs are clean. Fortunately, it's getting easier to find organic, cage-free eggs in many grocery stores. If you can get them fresh from a local farm, that's even better.

Can I have a piece of whole-wheat toast with my eggs?

You can have anything you want to have; our goal is not to be the Food Police or Diet Dictators but to simply point out the consequences of your choices. Sure, a single slice of bread isn't going to kill you. But the daily ingestion of lots of grains (toast at breakfast, a sandwich for lunch, bread basket at dinner) isn't doing you—or your waistline, or your heart—any good.

Commercially made bread is a high-GL food that generally has little nutrition, except for the paltry amount of vitamins that manufacturers throw back in to "enrich" it. It's not a great source of fiber, despite what you've been told, and there are no nutrients in bread that you can't get elsewhere. That said, both of us occasionally have a slice, particularly when it's homemade or rich in fiber—or particularly luscious. But we don't recommend bread as part of your daily diet, and it's certainly not part of the overall Smart Fat Solution blueprint for health.

You recommend steel-cut oats. Does that mean I can't have "regular" oatmeal? Steel-cut oats take so much longer to cook.

There are four kinds of oats in terms of cooking time: instant, or the kind you pour boiling water over and don't cook; quick-cooking, which take a few minutes on the stove or in the microwave; old-fashioned rolled oats, which take longer; and steel-cut oats, which take the longest, though we both believe they're worth the extra few minutes.

Instant oatmeal has very little fiber and is often presweetened with chemical additives, like artificial maple flavoring, which contain loads of added sugar (most often brown sugar, which is not any better than regular white table sugar). You might as well be eating a sugary kids' cereal if you eat the sweetened variety. Instant oats are pulverized, precooked, and processed so that they don't require cooking—you just pour hot water over them. Even if you go for the plain variety (and they are utterly bland, which is why manufacturers add phony flavor-ings), the manufacturers may have added sodium and other things you don't need. Convenient, yes, but they're a quick-release, high-GL carb compared with their more natural cousins, quick-cooking and old-fashioned oats.

Old-fashioned rolled oats have more fiber than instant oats (4 grams in a half cup, uncooked) and have a lower GL as well. *Quick-cooking oats* also have 4 grams of fiber, but because they are essentially smaller, chopped-up pieces of old-fashioned rolled oats, they may not have a lower GL than instant oats. Both taste a lot better than bland or artificially flavored, gummy instant oatmeal. Yes, they take longer to cook than instant oatmeal, but you can prepare rolled oats in the microwave in four to five minutes. By the time you've made a cup of coffee, the oatmeal is ready.

Steel-cut oats have the most fiber (5 grams in a ¼-cup, uncooked serving) and the lowest GL of all, which is why we like them the best. They also taste good—nutty, hearty, and genuinely oaty! Stir in some protein powder, top them with a handful of almonds or walnuts for some smart fat, add berries for more fiber and flavor, and they're a great way to start the day.

Steel-cut oats can cook in fewer than twenty minutes, or ten minutes if you're making a single serving. You can cook them on the stovetop, but they take only eight minutes in the microwave. If you prefer stove-top oats and want to shorten the cooking time, you can soak the oats in hot water (or almond milk) for about four minutes before you cook them, which softens them and shortens the cooking time. You can also get a head start and soak them overnight in water in your fridge.

If you prefer old-fashioned to steel-cut oats, go for it—just don't forget to add some protein powder, fresh fruit, and smart fat (walnuts or almonds taste great). If you are used to sweetening your oatmeal with lots of brown sugar and maple syrup, it's time to rethink that practice. Our recipe for steel-cut oatmeal is so delicious that you won't miss the sugar. If you can't bear eating oatmeal without a little sweetness in it, drizzle a small amount of organic honey or pure maple syrup to satisfy that "sweet tooth," but try to keep that drizzle to 1 teaspoon or less, especially now that you know about their effect on glycemic load! We hope that you'll find you won't need to sweeten, especially if you use enough berries.

What about sugar alternatives? Aren't "natural" ones better than artificial varieties?

Few subjects provoke more heated debate among nutritionists and health experts than the class of sugar alternatives called *artificial sweeteners.* You can find studies to back up nearly any position you take on these controversial substances. The reality is if you drink sodas daily, then you will lose a small amount of weight if you choose a diet soda over a regular soda, which has on average seven teaspoons of sugar. To make things even more complicated, artificial sweeteners are frequently used in diet beverages, and a whole body of emerging research suggests that artificial sweeteners in beverages confuse the appetite centers in the brain, accounting for the link between diet soda and obesity. Plus, artificial sweeteners appear to injure the healthy bacteria in our gut that provide us with powerful health benefits, so we don't think the long-term risks are worth the tiny benefit you may get from exchanging a sugar-loaded soda for an artificially sweetened one. But are "natural" sweeteners really any better? (See Chapter 3 where we discuss agave nectar, one of the worst offenders and most popularly hyped in recent years.)

Whether artificial or natural, sugar alternatives behave in the body just like regular table sugar, and there are plenty of reasons why—

despite the hype—they're no better than the white stuff (and may, in fact, be worse). Here are the ones you'll encounter most frequently.

Aspartame (found in NutraSweet and Equal): Aspartame is perhaps the most controversial and politicized of all the artificial sweeteners. Although plenty of industry-supported animal studies claim to show that aspartame is safe, many experts are not convinced. Russell Blaylock, for example, a retired neurosurgeon, has been outspoken in his criticism, calling aspartame a brain cell toxin. We think there are plenty of reasons to avoid this one. If we were ranking artificial sweeteners from good to bad, this would be at the very bottom of our list.

Sucralose (found in Splenda): Although sucralose is made from sugar, it is hardly natural. Sucralose is sucrose processed with chlorine, and there's evidence that it's passing through our bodies and winding up in our water systems. One research review published in the *Journal of Toxicology and Environmental Health* suggests that sucralose may cause a variety of harmful biological effects in the body. We'll take a pass.

Saccharin: Saccharin was the favorite artificial sweetener of our parents' generation until it got tagged with the reputation of causing bladder cancer in rats. Only in the past twenty years or so has it been found that saccharine is unlikely to have any negative effects in humans even at the highest concentrations—but we still can't shake the feeling that it just isn't good for you. Probably safe, but again, we'll take a pass.

What about natural sweeteners?—stevia, erythritol, and xylitol? Although we don't have any health concerns about using one to two servings per day of these three natural sweeteners, if you are trying to lose weight, stimulating your sweet taste buds without providing any calories will probably stimulate cravings and hunger. Each time you use these natural sweeteners, you will be compelled to eat more food within the next twenty-four hours to offset the noncaloric sweet your brain feels is its due.

The bottom line: For weight loss, we feel the best approach is to *avoid using sweeteners of any kind,* including items such as raw, unprocessed honey; maple syrup; and blackstrap molasses. These are real foods with actual minerals, but still, the body treats them the same way as it treats sugar.

If you are at your desired weight and are looking for healthier sweetener options, here's some more information.

Stevia is an herb that can be dried and used for sweetening. Commercially, it can be purchased in a powdered form. However, it has two shortcomings: It's not good for baking, and it can have a strong aftertaste that's reminiscent of licorice, a flavor that not everyone appreciates.

Erythritol is a sugar alcohol and is the main ingredient in the sweetener marketed as Truvia. It has no negative effects that we know of, although, as with all sugar alcohols, too much can cause diarrhea. Erythritol also stands up to heat and can be used in baking and in hot beverages like coffee. This is another acceptable choice.

Xylitol is a sugar alcohol naturally found in the fibers of many vegetables and fruits. It is frequently extracted from corn husks or birch. It has the property of helping to prevent the adhesion of bacteria onto mucous membranes, which is why it is so often used in what are touted as "healthy" chewing gums. Xylitol is much sweeter than sugar but contains only 2.4 calories per gram. If you want a natural sweetener, this is a healthy choice. But go easy, because like other sugar alcohols, too much can cause frequent trips to the bathroom.

What kind of milk can I put in my coffee?

Milk is one of the rare things that we do not agree on 100 percent. Jonny drinks only raw, whole milk (which is still available in California and through farm collectives); Steven is more cautious because of concerns about bacterial infections associated with raw milk (*Listeria, E. coli, Salmonella, Campylobacter*). But both of us agree that ordinary, homogenized, pasteurized milk (from factory-farmed cows) has the same problem as factory-farmed meat: Toxins are stored in the fat, so regular milk becomes a mean protein rather than a clean one. The solution? If you like milk, go with organic. Best of all, some brands now sell pasteurized organic milk from grass-fed cows. If you can find it, go for it. If you like milk in your coffee and can't find organic, do the next best thing and get skim milk. Or, learn to drink coffee black—it's actually pretty good!

And what about that creamy half-and-half? As long as it's organic, sure. You can also use organic (non-GMO) soy milk, unsweetened almond milk, and coconut milk.

But whatever you try with your coffee, *don't* put chemically enhanced creamers in it. They are basically embalming fluid. If you see multiple sugars and partially hydrogenated fats in the ingredients list, avoid them! As for those little individual containers of flavored "creamers"? Pure trans fat. Stay away!

What about making my own yogurt?

Why not? There are enormous joys and rewards involved in making your own food. So if you've got the time, patience, and interest, by all means go for it. But the same caveat applies here as everywhere else: Use the good stuff for ingredients. Remember the old saying about computers: Garbage in, garbage out. As with all food we prepare, it's all about the ingredients. Use organic milk and you'll have a terrific result. The benefits of naturally fermented foods like yogurt are legion. The naturally occurring probiotics support the immune system and may even give you an extra boost in your weight-loss efforts.

Do I need to eat breakfast before I exercise in the morning?

Some people do, some people don't. If your fasting blood sugar level is normal, it doesn't really matter if you eat breakfast before or after a workout. But if your fasting glucose level is elevated, there may be an advantage to eating before you work out so that you deplete the blood sugar stores in your muscles and you have more room to absorb calories you eat at lunchtime.

No one single strategy works for everyone under all circumstances. For the most part, we think eating breakfast is important and is a good "rule" for most people to follow. That's why we recommend it in this book. (That said, one of us—Jonny—plays tennis every morning on an empty stomach and then has breakfast afterwards. Steven has a protein-and-fiber-rich smoothie every morning on the way to the gym.) Our advice is to experiment with what works for you. For most people, that probably means eating breakfast, but when and how— we'll leave that up to you.

Lunch Smarts and Smart-Fat Snack Solutions

People in my office love to get together for lunch. I like to join them, but they always go to the worst greasy spoons. What can I order?

There are two problems with going out with co-workers who want to eat at the local junk food mecca. One obvious one is finding something healthy to eat. But the second problem is more daunting: going against the crowd. It's not easy, but it's far from impossible. You've got to privately take a stand for yourself and then decide how you're going to act. In the case of food, stick to your guns, don't make a big deal out of it, and eat what you think is right for you. (We offer the friendly advice that criticizing what other people are eating can annoy everyone at the table—and you're guaranteed not to win anyone over, even if what you're doing is healthier. You are usually much better off leading—quietly—by example.)

If asked, you might explain your health and weight-loss goals and how you're trying to get there; we'd hope that good friends and family members won't give you a hard time (and they may even get curious enough to try the Smart Fat Solution for themselves). As for people you don't know very well, expect a quip or two if you order a salad at a burger joint, but usually people are so involved in their own meals and conversation that they won't even notice what's on your plate.

If you find yourself at that greasy spoon, stick with salads and any vegetarian dishes—you won't find any clean protein there. Better yet, see whether you can subtly influence your colleagues to "trade up" on their dining choices. A growing number of fast-food chains (Chipotle, for example) are paying more attention to food quality, using organic and locally sourced ingredients, including some options from grass-fed or pasture-raised animals. As more and more people begin to realize that the food they're eating is making them sick, fat, tired, and depressed, the number of places offering alternatives to the usual fast-food junk is likely to grow.

I'm starving by the time I eat lunch. Why is that and what can I do?

Starving at lunch, low energy in the afternoon, falling asleep at dinner?—all these problems have one thing in common: They started before you noticed them.

People often ask us what they should do when they're starving at dinner or what they should "take" to get an energy boost in midafternoon. We think the problem probably began much earlier—at breakfast. If you're hungry by lunchtime, chances are that you didn't consume 20–30 grams of protein and 10–15 grams of fiber at breakfast. It's that simple. A high-protein, high-fiber (smart fat) breakfast will satisfy you for hours; most people won't feel hungry after a breakfast like that—at least not until lunchtime. This is why we like having a Smart Fat Shake for breakfast—it's so satisfying. You'll be comfortably hungry at lunchtime, but it's unlikely that you'll be starving.

Sometimes my work schedule means no lunch till early afternoon, and I get really hungry! Can I have a snack?

If you're having a hard time making it to lunch, snack on a full serving of protein and have some fiber. Take a few hardboiled eggs to work and some sliced veggies and hummus. If you just need a little something, go for fruit slices and nut butter or some almonds and a bit of dark chocolate. All of these snacks fall in line with the Smart Fat Solution.

Some people feel much better having a midmorning snack, and others can get by without one. If you need to fuel up between breakfast and lunch, no problem. Just make sure that you plan ahead for a snack that's smart fat–friendly. (By now you know the drill: ample

SMART-FAT YOUR LUNCH BOX

If you're used to bringing your lunch from home instead of heading for take-out, that's good news. That means you are used to being in control of what you eat when the clock strikes noon (or 1 . . . or 2 . . .). Now it's time to look in your lunch box and make sure it's smart-fat-friendly.

If your default lunch is a sandwich, a bag of chips, a cookie, and a can of something sweet, you already know what you need to do. It's time to break out of "sandwich jail." For the main course, consider any of our protein options, like sliced chicken or grass-fed beef. Include lots of crunchy veggies, a piece of fruit, and plenty of water. Add some dark chocolate for a treat.

You can also set aside some homemade soup or portions of leftover entrées from any of our recipes. If you have access to a microwave and fridge in your workplace, even better. Consider a bento-box type of lunch box, with individual containers to keep items fresh and separate. Pack ingredients for a breadless "wrap": sliced clean protein, flavorful sautéed veggies leftover from dinner, and some large lettuce leaves to wrap it all up. Delicious! Toss together ingredients for a smart fat salad— white beans, shrimp, and sliced grape tomatoes—with a dressing made from olive oil.

Assemble your lunch the night before. The secret to brown-bagging it the smart fat way is a bit of advanced planning—and making sure you have the right stuff in your kitchen!

protein, ample fiber, and a nice dollop of smart fat.) Be creative. Take some celery and almond butter to work, or a cup of shelled edamame, or a handful of pistachios. Get a "travel shaker" to mix up a simple protein shake when you're on the go. Find a protein bar that meets our standards—or whip one up yourself (you can find recipes on the Internet). Online, you can buy pemmican, a tasty mix of fat and protein that was first developed by North American Indians and used by explorers on polar expeditions. (See www.SmartFat.com for sources.) And it's a superior alternative to its modern fake-beef-jerky cousin, the notorious Slim Jim! If it's made from grass-fed beef, it's the perfect smart fat snack.

Find a snack solution that works for your lifestyle. If you eat as we suggest, keeping the principle of 5-5-10 servings in mind, you'll likely find that your between-meals hunger won't rule your life. But when you get the munchies, you can still feed that between-meals hunger—the smart fat way.

I love chips and I love dips—what can I eat instead?

Instead of chips, try satisfyingly crunchy jicama, radishes, carrots, cucumbers, bell peppers, celery, and raw veggies. Slice them into "chips" or sticks. They're easy to cut with a chef's knife, or if you want superthin slices, try an inexpensive mandoline slicer. Dip your healthy "chips" into hummus, guacamole, and bean dips for great snacks that combine veggie fiber with protein and smart fat, depending on what combinations you choose. You'll find some recipes in Chapter 10.

Is a protein bar a good snack option?

It is—at least in theory. The problem is finding one that meets our standards: no trans fat, a very low amount of sugar, a reasonable level of fiber (about 5 grams), some healthy fat, and a healthy amount of protein (about 10 grams). Few commercial protein bars meet these standards, however. There are some decent snack bars that meet *some* of these standards. If you can find one that meets most of our criteria, go for it.

(See www.SmartFat.com for our recommendations.) And if you're really ambitious, try making your own. You'll find lots of recipes for homemade protein bars on the Internet, particularly in the Paleo community.

You recommend dark chocolate as a snack. What should I look for?

Simple: Look for the highest percentage of cocoa you can reasonably stand. The higher the cocoa content, the more bitter the bar; an 82 percent cocoa bar may be sublimely healthy, but it might be hard to take when you're used to Hershey bars. The sweet spot for health and taste seems to be around 70–75 percent cocoa. (Dark chocolate with more than 70 percent cocoa, and consequently less sugar, has been shown to lower blood pressure; but add more sugar, and the blood pressure benefits disappear.) And don't limit yourself to merely eating your dark chocolate—you can drink it, too! If you're a coffee drinker, enjoy the taste (and health benefits) of a tablespoon of unsweetened cocoa stirred into your morning coffee. Chocolate and coffee are a terrific combination. (You may notice a bit of undissolved cocoa residue in the bottom of your coffee cup—but no worries, you'll still get its benefits.)

Cocoa is where all-important health-enhancing cocoa flavanols are found. The less cocoa, the fewer flavanols. Milk chocolate has very few; white chocolate has none. Organic high-cocoa chocolate bars are also less likely to be made with fillers and extra sugar, making them an ideal choice for a smart fat snack.

I'm willing to cut the "J" from my PB&J sandwich, and I'll even cut the bread, but I still love peanut butter. What should I look for when I shop?

Hey, who doesn't love peanut butter? We certainly do. But we don't love the trans fat–laden, sugar-enriched commercial kinds that we all grew up with. These days it's not hard to find a grocery store where you can grind your own peanuts (and other nuts) and turn them into healthy butters. When you do this, the only ingredient is peanuts—with perhaps a touch of salt. And there are plenty of organic, healthy brands that don't add sugar and hydrogenated oils. It's no longer hard to find a brand that has a very short ingredients list: that is, peanuts and salt.

That said, try expanding your palate. Almond butter is a terrific alternative to peanut butter, and in some ways it's even healthier. (Almonds have a better "fat profile," in our opinion, and aren't as allergenic as peanuts and peanut products.) And why not try some tahini?—which is basically a "nut" butter except that it's made from sesame seeds. It's versatile and delicious!

Dinner Smarts

I love pasta but have resolved to cut back so I can follow the Smart Fat Solution. Does this mean it's off the table forever?

Nothing's "off the table" forever if you don't want it to be. We don't want to turn you into a food robot. We all run into situations where we're presented with scrumptious dishes that are a sensual and culinary delight, even though they might not qualify for a "best in class" in the food sweepstakes. But what would life be without the possibility of a bit—emphasis on *a bit*—of recreational eating once in a while? We don't want to forbid these foods but to make you aware of their effects (on your blood sugar, on inflammation, on your waistline, etc.). Pasta isn't a staple diet item for either of us, but that doesn't mean we don't occasionally succumb to the chef's special homemade lobster ravioli at a local family-owned trattoria. We just don't do it very often.

And think about Italy, where pasta is served as a first course before the entrée (protein!) and usually with a portion of deliciously prepared vegetables, beans, or a green salad. Pasta there is always cooked al dente (which lowers its GL), with a heavenly freshly made sauce and likely a sprinkle of freshly grated cheese, too. Take a lesson from the Italians and enjoy pasta (a small portion) as part of a varied, healthy, and tasty meal.

SIZING UP YOUR FOOD—WITHOUT A SCALE

Here's a list that will help you get a visual handle on portion sizes. With regard to a "handful," we're aware that a smaller person has smaller hands than a larger person. Not all handfuls are created equal, and neither are our bodies. But here's a general rule: Larger people will be fine with their naturally larger handfuls, and smaller people will be satisfied with their smaller handfuls.

1 ounce of nuts = a handful

3–4 ounces of protein = a deck of cards

8 ounces of protein = two decks of cards or a thin paperback book

1 ounce of hard cheese = one domino (or four dice, or a 1-inch cube)

1 cup cooked grains = a tennis ball

1 medium-size piece of fruit = a tennis ball

2 tablespoons of nut butter = a golf ball

1 serving (½ cup) of cooked pasta = a rounded handful

Should I give up the bread basket?

Unless something special is being celebrated, just about everyone should give up the bread basket. You don't need empty flour calories sending your blood sugar levels sky-rocketing and disrupting your hormones and metabolism. Think of bread like birthday cake—it's something you should save for special occasions.

What about just going gluten-free?

Going gluten-free is different from "giving up the bread basket."

Gluten sensitivity is poorly understood and vastly more serious than an ordinary food intolerance. Let's use lactose intolerance—the most common of the food intolerances—as a comparison.

Lactase is the enzyme you need to digest milk sugar (lactose), and when you don't have lactase, consuming milk, ice cream, and other dairy products makes you gassy and bloated. For some people it can also result in painful abdominal cramps. But other than some annoying symptoms, eating dairy won't kill you. Gluten, however, is a different story.

Gluten is a protein found in wheat, rye, and barley. Every time you eat one of these grains—in whatever form—you consume gluten. Your immune system "sees" the gluten and treats it like a foreign invader, making antibodies that attack the gluten foreigner. By itself, this wouldn't be such a bad thing—except that many of these antibodies get confused and attack not just the gluten, but your body's own tissues. These antibodies can wreak havoc on your gut lining, joints, thyroid, sinuses, and even your brain.

Gluten sensitivity is essentially a form of autoimmune disease. If gluten-sensitive people eat gluten even once, they may find their immune systems attacking their tissues for the next twenty to thirty days. The symptoms may persist for many weeks because the antibody attack can be relentless.

Symptoms of gluten sensitivity include gastrointestinal issues, such as bloating, gas, and abdominal pain; nutrient deficiencies; brain fog; attention deficit disorder (ADD); anxiety; achy joints; sinus congestion; fatigue; eczema and skin rashes; and weight gain and resistance to weight loss. You could have all of these symptoms, or only one or two. Anyone with similar chronic, unexplained symptoms deserves testing or a gluten-free trial. Many doctors order an outdated blood test for gluten, so it's important to make sure that you get the right test.

If you are gluten-sensitive, your immune system is attacking your own tissues. If you have celiac disease, your immune system is attacking your gut and damaging your small intestine. Many people have the mistaken idea that if they have an intestinal biopsy and they don't have celiac disease, then they can eat gluten. But this isn't the case. Gluten sensitivity can exacerbate or lead to all kinds of problems, including multiple sclerosis, as these antibodies can impact your brain. Plus, gluten can make you feel groggy, achy—just all around awful. People with gluten sensitivity are very inflamed, which slows their metabolism and promotes weight gain.

Gluten sensitivity is a life-threatening problem. Please don't confuse it with something that is merely annoying, like lactose intolerance. For more information on gluten sensitivity, gluten testing, and gluten-free living, visit our website at www.SmartFat.com.

> ### You allow some wine with dinner (after Phase 1). What about alcohol in general? How does that fit with the Smart Fat Solution?

Drinking one serving of alcohol daily has numerous benefits. Alcohol improves blood sugar control, increases insulin sensitivity, enhances cholesterol profiles, decreases the risk for having a stroke or heart attack, aids digestion, and even decreases the risk of food poisoning. But with alcohol, the dose is very important. One serving daily, medically speaking, is better than none; but two servings daily have no added benefit. And three servings daily increases overall health risk, especially for cancer. At this level of consumption, alcohol actually worsens blood sugar and blood pressure. And drinking four or more servings every day? Yikes! That isn't just bad for your physical health, it's also destructive to your social and work lives and may indicate a deeper personal issue that needs addressing.

Part of the reason that too much alcohol is associated with increased cancer risk is because alcohol uses up *folate,* an important member of the B-vitamin family. Without folate, cancer risks increase. In fact, in the famous Nurses' Health Study (one of the longest-running studies on women's health ever undertaken), one or more drinks a day increased the risk for breast cancer—but only in women who were deficient in folate (folic acid). So if you indulge in moderate alcohol, make sure you get your B vitamins!

And remember that there's nothing wrong with not drinking any alcohol. (One of us—Jonny—hasn't had an alcoholic beverage since the early 1980s.) For many people, the concept of "moderation" just doesn't decode in their brain, so they shouldn't use alcohol at all. Please don't think you *need* to add alcohol for the benefits noted. You can get those benefits other ways besides drinking.

Which is the best type of alcohol to consume?

All forms of alcohol—wine, hard liquor, and beer—have benefits if limited to one serving daily. From Steven's perspective, wine makes food taste better, so it's his first choice for an alcoholic beverage. There are also some biochemical and laboratory results that clearly favor wine. In our opinion, the best choice is red wine, followed by white wine, beer, and finally hard liquor, which inflicts the most damage to your liver. Red wine has several benefits, including being an aid to digestion. It also has an anticlotting benefit and contains an important health-promoting flavonoid called *resveratrol* (see Chapter 8).

Unless you are ultra-disciplined and can keep your alcohol intake to a maximum of one serving daily, Steven suggests you skip alcohol use at least two to three days per week.

I love your recipes, but does everything need to be organic?

Fresh, local, organic food, direct from the farm to your table, is always best. But this is very far from a perfect world, and we believe in choosing our battles wisely.

Every year the Environmental Working Group—a nonprofit consumer advocacy group—uses USDA data about pesticide residues in produce to come up with an annual list they call the Dirty Dozen—the most contaminated produce. Apples, peaches, nectarines, and strawberries have been at the top in recent years. When you're shopping for foods on this list, look for the organic versions. You can download a free app at EWG's website (www.ewg.org) and turn your smartphone into a "smart fat phone." EWG also compiles a list called the Clean Fifteen, which includes produce items that have the least amount of pesticide residue. Recent "clean" picks include avocados, sweet peas, pineapples, and cabbage. There's less of a need to purchase organic versions of the Clean Fifteen.

We also recommend that you add milk, meat, poultry, and coffee to your shopping list of organic items. Coffee is one of the most sprayed crops on the planet, and you already know how we feel about toxic meat and milk!

I like salty foods, but I hear so much about the problem of too much sodium in our diets. What do you recommend?

For your overall health, we clearly prefer that you focus on the smart fat principle of 5-5-10 servings daily rather than salt and sodium. Saltiness is one of the primary tastes we humans are drawn to, and adding a little bit of salt to foods makes them taste better. The critical phrase here is "a little bit."

There are about 2,400 milligrams of sodium in 1 teaspoon of salt— about the amount that health authorities recommend as the daily upper limit for sodium consumption. The problem is that most of the sodium we consume doesn't come from the salt shaker. It comes from processed foods, canned soups, prepared meals, and foods we eat in restaurants. The "little bit" of salt we add to unprocessed food is just a drop in the bucket.

For most people salt isn't an issue of life or death. That said, if you have high blood pressure, you could experiment and see whether limiting your salt intake reduces your blood pressure.

It's worth noting, too, that salt and potassium have an ideal ratio in the human diet, much like omega-3 and omega-6 fats. Many health professionals have pointed out that the problem in our diet may not be just that we consume too much sodium; we also may be consuming not enough potassium. Potassium is found in most vegetables and many fruits, so when you eat the smart fat way, you'll be eating a potassium-rich diet.

You'll notice that most of our recipes use about ⅛ to ¼ teaspoon salt per person, which is ample to stimulate your taste buds. This meets national recommendations to keep salt intake in the 2,000 to 2,400 daily range. But your taste buds will be even happier if you stimulate all of the five basic tastes: salty, sour, sweet, bitter, and umami (a Japanese word meaning a pleasant savory or meaty taste). The challenge with cooking is to stimulate all your taste buds—as that makes your food taste fantastic.

So, what if at the end of the day I still like a low-fat eating plan and I've done well on it in the past?

Both of us used to be advocates of low-fat eating plans, but we have abandoned this approach for the reasons we mention in Chapter 1. If

SMART MOVE: PREP YOUR BEANS TO REDUCE LECTIN (AND TOOTING)

We love nutrient-packed beans and legumes as part of the Smart Fat Solution, but we know that some of you may be intolerant to proteins known as *lectins* found in these foods. (The 10 percent or so of people who are lectin-intolerant experience a strong reaction when they eat beans and legumes, including symptoms such as bloating and diarrhea.) We're not talking about the "tooting" that beans are famously associated with—we're talking about real gastrointestinal distress. If you fall into this group, it's possible to greatly reduce irritating lectins in beans and legumes by "sprouting" them before you cook them. It's simple to do.

To sprout most beans, soak them overnight and then rinse them in the morning and soak again for six to eight hours. By the time you get home from work, they're ready to be rinsed one more time and cooked in fresh water. (Note: Though this is called "sprouting," you don't actually have to see a sprout forming; soaking the bean is what removes the lectins.)

you have had personal success with a low-fat eating plan and you want to stick with that, *our 5-5-10 message remains the same:* Choose smart fat (five servings), add clean protein (five servings), and make sure you get enough fiber (ten servings) every day. Some people can do well with less fat in their diets, but we don't think you should go lower than three to four servings of smart fat per day. A higher carb diet should be fine—as long as you choose low-GL carbs and leave out grains and starches whenever possible.

Studies have shown that genetic makeup can affect how people lose weight: Some do better with fewer carbs and more protein and fat; others are better off with a more "Mediterranean" (balanced) eating plan. Some do better with a low-fat diet. To find out whether

---

For those of you with less serious problems—that is, you're concerned about the noise that this "musical fruit" is renowned for making—soaking beans, rinsing them well, and cooking them in fresh water, not the water you soak them in, helps to reduce flatulence, which is most common in people who aren't used to eating beans. (The old rhyme "Beans, beans, the musical fruit, the more you eat, the more you toot" is actually due for a rewrite—because the more you eat, the more you get used to them, and the *less* you toot!) Rinse canned beans completely, as well.[†]

Beans and legumes are among the healthiest foods to ever come out of the earth, and you'll see a lot of them in the pages of this book because they do "triple duty": They are full of fiber, nutrients, and protein. Though canned varieties are convenient, cooking your own is worth it (and dried beans are much cheaper than canned).

[†] It's a myth that you have to soak dried beans overnight before you cook them. Soaking does cut cooking time by up to half an hour, but there's no cook's rule that they *must* be soaked. If you want to avoid the buildup of the compounds that cause flatulence, however, soaking beans properly helps. If you don't remember to soak overnight but you want them for tonight's dinner, try a quick "hot soak." Bring rinsed, picked-over beans to a boil in enough cold water to cover them; boil for two minutes, and then let them soak for at least an hour. This will reduce the amount of oligosaccharides, a type of carbohydrate that causes gas.

people have a genetic advantage for success with one eating plan over another, Steven offers genetic testing at his clinic that looks at genotypes and which eating plan may be best for you.

I've had my smart fat breakfast, lunch, and dinner—plus I smart-fatted all my snacks! I'm pretty sure I stuck to the plan, but I wonder whether I should keep a food diary.

Keeping a food diary takes work and is inconvenient, and frankly, most of us don't like being confronted with the sometimes-ugly truth about what we actually eat every day. But, there's no getting around it: Keeping a food diary can be your best friend on the weight-loss journey. One 2008 study showed that keeping a food diary can *double* a person's weight loss. That's impressive! A 2011 review of fifteen studies focused on "self-monitoring" during weight loss found that there was a significant association between self-monitoring and weight loss. And more than half of all the participants in the National Weight Control Registry—which tracks people who have lost at least 30 pounds and kept it off for at least a year—regularly keep food diaries.

If you follow the Smart Fat Solution closely, especially if you make use of the Phase 1 and Phase 2 meal plans and recipes, you won't need a food diary. But you're probably going to go "off the reservation" at some point, and you may even find that you've drifted a few pounds away from your target. That's where a food diary comes in. Keeping a record of what you eat—even for a few days—can accomplish a lot. It's an eye opener, and it helps you track your progress. It also keeps you mindful of what you're eating. It's very hard to eat without thinking when you've made a promise to yourself to write everything down!

Here's a way to use a food diary as part of the Smart Fat Solution. Try keeping one for up to three days when you start Phase 1—particularly so you can track your 5-5-10 intake of smart fat, protein, and fiber. Then, try it again for a few days when you're in Phase 2 as a way to make sure that you're still within the smart fat recommendations. Try it one more time when you are past Day 31—again, just to make sure that you're aware of what you're eating and that you're still hitting the 5-5-10 mark. Make the diary as simple or as detailed as you want; do whatever works for you, but at the very least, try it when you first start the Thirty-Day Plan and then as a check later on.

If you go this route, you don't have to keep a diary forever. Jonny once went on a monthlong journey to track every single morsel he put into his mouth. He tracked protein grams, carb grams, fat grams, calories—all of it—and also kept note of his exercise habits just for good measure. At the end, he had learned a great deal about what his body needed to lose, gain, or maintain weight. He never repeated the experiment, but the knowledge he gained during that month was invaluable. Steven does a three-day food diary analysis at least once every year, and he learns something important about his nutrient intake from it every time.

Food diaries can help you snap out of a plateau funk or bring you back to eating right if you slip up from time to time. Don't eat right just to keep a food diary; keep a food diary to eat right!

Should I throw away my scale, or weigh myself regularly?

The ordinary bathroom scale is an object that inspires terror in a lot of people—but it shouldn't. The scale is a good way of getting feedback from the universe. It's a reality check, and it tells you when it's time for a course correction.

The trick to using the scale in a healthy, productive way is not to give it too much power. It's just providing you with a number. It's just a way of telling you how you're doing, what direction you're heading, and whether you need to make any modifications. It should not tyrannize you or define you, and don't ever think that the number you see is the ultimate arbiter of your health, your well-being, or even how good you look. *You* are in charge, not this thing you are standing on.

Here are four tips for using a body-weight scale in a productive way:

1. Always use the same scale.
2. Always weigh yourself in the morning.
3. Always weigh yourself naked.
4. Always weigh yourself before you eat.

Jonny uses what he calls "the 4-pound rule." If he gets more than 4 pounds away from his goal weight, he goes back to a more stringent way of eating (such as Phase 1 of the Thirty-Day Plan). You never want to be the guy who has a high school reunion, puts on the tux he hasn't worn in years, and "suddenly" realizes that he's gained 25 pounds without noticing. Use the scale! It will help you stay conscious. Make it your friend and ally, not your enemy. Think of it as just another way to get important information about what's working for you and what's not.

We have one caveat, however: An ordinary scale won't tell you anything about body composition, which is an important metric when you're trying to lose weight. Remember: You want to lose *body fat,* not *muscle.* (People who lose weight without preserving muscle often find that they become "skinny fat.") Fortunately, a number of higher-end home scales now tell you your body fat percentage as well as your weight. These body fat percentages are reliable within 2 and 4 percent (as they depend upon hydration), and they give you a good idea of what direction you're going in. You can purchase a bioelectrical impedance (BEI) scale for less than $100. You can also find high-level BEI scales in some doctors' offices, gyms, and spas.

If you truly want to use a scale to track your progress, ditch your old-school bathroom scale and replace it with a BEI model (see www .SmartFat.com for recommendations). We think it's worth it if you're a scale-user. (A note on hydration: Being more hydrated can change your body fat percentage numbers by 1–2 percent, so when you're tracking improvements using a BEI scale, ignore any changes unless they are more than 2 percent.)

My weight loss was moving along at a great pace, but I've reached that plateau and now it has stopped. What can I do?

In our combined fifty-five years of practice, neither of us has ever seen a person successfully lose weight over time without encountering the dreaded "plateau"—that point in the weight-loss journey where weight loss seems to stop dead in its tracks. This plateau is frustrating for everybody, but you can do a couple of things about it.

First is to think about your weight loss differently. Your weight—or more correctly, your body fat percentage—is like the stock market. You can't pay attention to every change that happens on an hourly graph of stock market activity—you'd go crazy. What's important, with stocks and with weight loss, is the *overall direction* of the graph. The little daily dips and surges that happen throughout the day in the stock market don't matter very much if you look at the big picture and see that over time the stock market is generally going up. Similarly, your weight can fluctuate by a couple of pounds from day to day, but what's important is what's happening *over the long haul,* that is, that it's generally going down. Plateaus are a part of the weight-loss journey. The trick is not to be defeated by them but to plan for them and not be surprised (or derailed) when they happen.

One common reason for plateauing: If you are following our recommendations, *your fat mass will decrease and your muscle mass will increase,* so your total weight won't change. This doesn't mean that you're plateauing; you're actually doing a great job because you want more muscle mass to burn fat! But still, you might get hung up on the number on that bathroom scale. Don't! Instead, measure your fat mass and lean mass and track them separately (you'll need a BEI scale to do this).

That said, other forces are often at work that can contribute to (or cause) plateaus, and if you're stuck for a while at the same weight and nothing seems to be working, it might be time to consider some of these. For example, many patients in Steven's clinic have a test to measure basal metabolic rate (BMR), especially if they have any challenges losing weight. BMR is the rate at which you burn calories when you are at rest.

Steven's clinic also offers genetic testing. Both genetic testing and metabolic rate can be important pieces of information when you're setting out to modify a diet. (For example, some people with a certain variant of the gene that may be correlated with obesity actually do better with a lower smart fat diet!)

Two other factors that can cause, or prolong, plateaus are food intolerances and toxins. If you're eating a food to which you are sensitive, your body may be responding by making a lot of inflammatory chemicals that can interfere with a smoothly running metabolism, not to mention burning fat. (Undiagnosed food sensitivities are a frequent cause of weight-loss plateaus.) So if you hit a prolonged weight-loss plateau, consider trying a food allergy elimination diet. (Visit our website at www.SmartFat.com for details.)

Another thing to consider is that when you lose a lot of fat, you release a lot of toxins. While that fat is melting off your hips, butt, and thighs, it's also, unfortunately, releasing a bunch of stored toxins into your bloodstream. These toxins lower your metabolism (the rate at which you burn calories), and they make you feel grumpy and sick. If you've been eating dirty fat and mean protein for years, guess what? You're probably loaded with toxins, and when those babies get released into your system, all hell can break loose.

Though there's no scientifically accurate agreed-upon test for measuring toxins, you can safely assume that if you've been eating the Standard American Diet of mean protein and dirty fat, you've got toxins galore in your body, and they block your calorie-burning ability dramatically. If toxins are holding you back from losing weight, it might be time to add some detox supplements that can help your liver do its job of clearing them from your system. The ones we like are milk thistle (900 milligrams a day), N-acetylcysteine (NAC; 600 milligrams a day), curcumin (500–1,000 milligrams a day), and selenium

(400 micrograms a day). Your total intake of selenium from food and supplements should not exceed 400 mcg. Keep in mind that your multivitamin may have 100–200 mcg of selenium. (See Chapter 8 for more on supplements.)

A low-tech solution to plateaus is as simple as it is elegant: Drink more water. The formula we both like for weight loss is to take your weight, divide by two, and drink that number of ounces of water every day. (So if you weigh 150 pounds, you should be drinking 75 ounces every day, or a little more than nine 8-ounce glasses of water.) Meanwhile, try sweating more. Exercise may not be the most effective way to lose weight (that honor goes to diet), but it's one of the best ways to assure that you continue to hold on to your gains. Try upping your activity level or intensity.

Probably the best advice of all when it comes to plateaus is also the hardest to follow: Be patient. Plateaus are a fact of life on the weight-loss journey. And they're not the *end* of that journey—they're just a minor obstacle in the road.

PART THREE

Beyond Diet: Smart for Life

CHAPTER 8

Smart Supplements

WHEN YOU SMART-FAT YOUR DIET, you're going to be eating a wide variety of nutritionally dense foods. A smart fat diet will provide plenty of essential vitamins, minerals, omega-3 fats, and other healthful compounds that will help you to turn back the clock on aging, improve your energy, shrink your waistline, and even improve your love life. We're betting you'll even see an increased sharpness in memory and thinking.

So, you might be wondering: If all this food in the Smart Fat Solution is so great, why the need for nutritional supplements? Don't experts tell us that if we eat a healthy diet we can get all the nutrients we need from food?

Well, yes, they do.

And they're wrong.

If we all lived in a perfect environment where crops were grown in nutrient-rich soil, where all our food was organic, where we ate a wide variety of plant foods every day, where the air was clean and the water was pure, and our stress levels were low and we all lived south of Atlanta and got one to two hours of sunshine while dressed in a bathing suit—then sure, we could probably get all the basic vitamins and minerals from our food, our earth, and our sun. But none of us lives at that address.

Because of how we grow and produce our food today, we've processed and engineered much of the "good stuff" right out of our food supply. Modern farming practices and soil cultivation have resulted in lower levels of certain minerals like magnesium and selenium in the very soil in which plants are grown. As for our exposure to healthy clean air and sunlight, few of us live in cities or towns (or even undeveloped areas) where every breath of air is pollutant-free. And with increasing use of sunscreen—a must to prevent skin cancer—we don't get enough exposure to sunlight, which helps our bodies produce must-have vitamin D.

So, can we get enough vitamins and minerals through diet? With the Smart Fat Solution you will most definitely meet—and exceed—the minimum nutritional requirements for the major nutrients experts agree upon. But if you truly want optimal health—if you want to build upon that healthy diet and supercharge your health for the long haul—then think of supplements as a high-tech delivery system for the nutrients your body needs to thrive.

What About Those "Recommended Daily Allowances," or RDAs?

We are not huge fans of the recommended daily allowances. Most people aren't aware that the RDAs were designed to answer the question: What amount of this particular vitamin will prevent a disease related to nutritional deficiency in 97 percent of the population? In other words, "How much vitamin C does the average human need to prevent scurvy?" or "How much vitamin D does that person need to prevent rickets?" RDAs were developed during World War II as part of the dietary recommendations for soldiers and others who were living on rations. They aren't—and never were—a good measure of what nutrients we need for optimal health, and there is a vast difference between the minimum amount we need to avoid a specific vitamin-deficiency-triggered disease and the optimal amount we should have for overall excellent health.

Think of it this way. If you want to prevent rickets, make sure you meet the RDA for vitamin D. If you want to reduce heart disease, improve brain function, lower your risk of cancer, stop bone loss, and do countless other things to prevent accelerated aging, then go for the optimal amount—which is about 300 percent more than the RDA! We're going to tell you how to get that amount—and that's where supplements come in.

All Supplements Are *Not* Created Equal

Knowing where your food comes from is an essential part of smart fat eating, and it's exactly the same thing with supplements. If your fish oil comes from wild salmon caught in pristine Alaskan waters, is made in small batches, is molecularly distilled and tested for impurities, that's one thing. If your generic (and suspiciously inexpensive) "fish oil" comes from unidentified, unregulated sources, that's quite another. You could be supplementing with a product made from toxic fish from polluted waters. With supplements, as with food, quality matters.

From time to time, a study will come out showing that many commercial supplements do not contain what their label says they do. For example, in 2015, *Scientific Reports* noted that only 10 percent of fish oil products marketed in New Zealand contained the amount of eicosapentaenoic acid (EPA) and docosahexaenoic acid (DHA), important omega-3 fats, as listed on the label. Even worse, 83 percent of the commercial fish oil products tested showed unacceptable levels of oxidation, which is a fancy way of saying the products were rancid.

ConsumerLab.com is a kind of watchdog for the supplement industry, performing independent testing on a wide range of commercially available vitamins, minerals, and other nutritional supplements. Sadly, they frequently find evidence that what's in the bottle doesn't match what's on the label. In one recent test, they found "defects" in nearly 40 percent of multivitamins. ConsumerLab.com has also found probiotics that don't have the number of live organisms as claimed on the label; magnesium supplements with misleading labels, including one that had only 45 percent of the magnesium claimed on the label; and weight-loss supplements with all kinds of garbage in them.

Because physicians are *not* normally trained in nutrition (many physicians have had at most a four-hour elective in nutrition during medical school), they often start out being inherently suspicious of supplements. Findings like these only tend to make them even more skeptical, causing many of them to suggest that their patients avoid supplements altogether.

Unfortunately, that's a shortsighted (and uninformed) approach. More than 80 percent of Americans are nutritionally deficient to such a degree that their health is affected and their aging process is accelerated. The answer to the quality problem is not to stop taking supplements—it's to take *better quality* supplements. Unfortunately, you're rarely going to find them at your regular grocery store, "big box" stores, or local pharmacy.

Brands we take ourselves (and recommend to our family and friends) are usually purchased from a licensed medical provider or a company they recommend online. Steven's clinic offers products from Designs for Health, Thorne Research, Metagenics, ProThera, and Xymogen. Jonny offers his clients products from Designs for Health, Integrative Therapeutics, Vital Nutrients, Pure Encapsulations, Euro-Pharma, Pharmax, and other brands usually available through health practitioners, select online stores, and the occasional specialty pharmacy. Jonny also recommends some widely available mass market brands and has found a number of them—Barlean's, Reserveage, Terry Naturally, Ocean Blue, Jarrow, and Garden of Life—that meet his exacting standards for quality. (Full disclosure: Jonny is a partner in Rockwell Nutrition, an online vitamin store that carries only premium brands.)

You can shop for supplements confidently if you follow a few basic tips:

- *Buy products manufactured in FDA-approved facilities.* Look for products produced under conditions certified as following "current good manufacturing practices" (CGMP). The FDA closely regulates and audits drug-GMP facilities in the United States on a regular schedule.
- *Buy from the best.* Many licensed medical professionals, including physicians, nutritionists, and chiropractors, offer dietary supplements for sale. If you're purchasing from a reputable healthcare provider, the product is more likely to be of high quality and safe.
- *Check the date.* You can buy quality products online, but confirm the expiration date; sometimes expired supplements, including those from reputable manufacturers that find their way into the marketplace, are sold at a steep discount for this reason. You wouldn't eat bad fish—and you shouldn't take expired fish oil, or anything else that is past its sell-by date.
- *Don't bargain-hunt.* An integrative medical doctor friend of Jonny's used to have a framed poster in his New York City office that said, "There are three things you shouldn't bargain-shop for: Parachutes, tattoos and vitamins." A cost-saving option in any of these categories may save you money up front, but in the long run? Not so much. If you see a product at a price that seems too good to be true, it probably is.

Remember, dietary supplements are exactly what they're billed as—supplements. They are *supplemental* to a good diet and a healthy lifestyle, not a substitute for them. Used smartly, they can provide therapeutic doses of important nutrients that are difficult to get from food, at least in the optimal doses. They can also provide good insurance that your body has all the micronutrients it needs every day. The trick, as with everything else, is to be smart about how to use them.

What We Recommend and Why

We're both big believers in the concept of biochemical individuality, which basically means that *everybody's different.* Though all of us share certain characteristics as humans, each of us is metabolically, physiologically, psychologically, hormonally, and biochemically unique. "One size fits all" simply has no place in diet, exercise, or nutritional supplementation. What follows are the supplements both of us have taken—but that doesn't mean we think you should necessarily take the exact same things. We recommend that you work with a healthcare provider who is knowledgeable in nutrition to come up with an individualized plan that's right for you.

At a minimum, we strongly recommend you take a multivitamin and that you meet our recommendations for magnesium, vitamin K, fish oil (omega-3), and vitamin D. We also like probiotics, as human studies show good clinical evidence for their benefit, as well as a few others

---

THE THERAPEUTIC GOODS ADMINISTRATION: THE "GOLD STANDARD" OF SUPPLEMENTS

Australia, Germany, France, and many other countries have quality supplement standards that far exceed those in the United States. For a U.S. manufacturer to sell its products in Australia, for example, the manufacturer must meet the exacting standards of Australia's Therapeutic Goods Administration (TGA). We mention the TGA certification because it is an extremely high-quality standard that we would like to see more manufacturers achieve. The fact that a brand does not have TGA certification doesn't mean it's not any good, since many excellent brands are not distributed internationally and therefore have not sought out TGA certification. But you can be very sure that brands that *do* have TGA certification, such as Thorne Research and Metagenics, are formulated with the highest quality ingredients and meet the strictest quality standards.

that we'll explain below. Finally, we also suggest that if you want to lose weight you either drink green tea or take EGCG (epigallocatechin gallate), a beneficial compound extracted from green tea.

Multivitamins

If you want to meet some basic vitamin and mineral needs all at once, a multivitamin is a great place to start. However, no single multivitamin will have enough of *every* vitamin and mineral that your body needs. For example, some minerals, such as calcium and magnesium, are made up of molecules that are literally too big to fit into a multivitamin, at least in doses that would be meaningful. If you've ever wondered why some tablets and capsules look like "horse pills," it's usually because the molecular structure of the active ingredients is naturally large, complex, and bulky. Ideally, pills shouldn't be too big to swallow comfortably. That's why the "serving size" on some high-quality multivitamins is often two to three pills (or more).

One of the reasons your personal physician may *not* recommend a multivitamin is that most multivitamin studies to date have been done using multivitamins with very poor-quality ingredients that neither of us would recommend. Studies using a poor-quality multivitamin did not decrease the risk of heart attacks and strokes, and these no-benefit studies received a very high level of coverage in the medical literature. For reasons we fail to understand, researchers designing large-scale multivitamin studies in the past have insisted that the ingredients combined had to be ultra-cheap (usually as low as pennies per day), which obviously limits their effectiveness. Furthermore, getting people to volunteer for a multivitamin study is very difficult. A study published in the prestigious *Journal of the American Medical Association* showed that people enrolling for multivitamin studies ate vastly better than average Americans in the first place, which greatly limited the benefit that would have been shown for the average American.

Yet, despite the poor-quality ingredients used, national multivitamin studies have revealed more benefits than your doctor may want to admit. Solid studies have shown that taking even a poor-quality multivitamin daily decreases your risk for cancer and decreases damage to your DNA. We believe the benefits of taking a high-quality multivitamin greatly outweigh any risk, and we highly recommend that you take a multivitamin daily.

Some ingredients suggest that a supplement is being made with inferior ingredients, similar to those used in the national studies noted. When you see these, start looking for a better quality supplement brand. Here are a few examples:

- Beta carotene ➔ *Instead, look for mixed carotenoids.*
- Alpha tocopherol ➔ *Instead, look for mixed tocopherols.*
- Magnesium oxide ➔ *Instead, look for magnesium citrate, magnesium glycinate, magnesium malate, or a chelated form of magnesium.*
- Folic acid ➔ *Instead, look for mixed folates.* The most absorbable and metabolically active kind of folate is 5-methyltetrahydrofolate.
- Zinc-to-copper ratio > 10–20 ➔ *Instead, look for a zinc-to-copper ratio that is at least 20 or more.* Copper and zinc that aren't in the right balance can increase the risk for cancer. The fact is that you can get all the copper you need from eating healthy food, so if your supplement has zinc and omits copper, that's just fine (like the foods on the Smart Fat plan). Make sure you have at least 20–25 parts zinc for each part copper.

We include a chart from Steven's clinic outlining guidelines for ingredients in an ideal multivitamin. Not many brands contain all of these nutrients in the exact doses and forms listed, but this chart can still serve as a good template for you to use when evaluating any multivitamin.

RECOMMENDED INGREDIENTS FOR A SMART FAT MULTIVITAMIN		
VITAMIN, MINERAL, COMPOUND	RECOMMENDED FORM	DOSAGE (daily)*
Vitamin A	Palmitate	2,000 IU
Carotenoids	Mixed carotenoids	3,000 IU
Vitamin D	Cholecalciferol (D3)	2,000 IU
Vitamin E	Mixed tocopherols	50 mg (total)
Vitamin K		500 mcg (total)
	Vitamin K1	300 mcg
	Vitamin K2	200 mcg
Vitamin C	Ascorbic acid	250 mg
Thiamin (vitamin B1)	Thiamin HCl	50 mg
Riboflavin (vitamin B2)	Riboflavin 5-phosphate	12 mg
Niacin (vitamin B3)	Niacinamide	80 mg
Pyridoxine (vitamin B6)	Pyridoxal-5-phosphate	20 mg
Folic acid (folates)	Mixed folates, including 5-methyltetrahydrofolate	400 mcg
Vitamin B12	Methylcobalamin	500 mcg
Biotin (vitamin B7)		500 mcg
Vitamin B5	Calcium pantothenate	45 mg
Boron	Bororganic glycine	2 mg
Copper	Copper glycinate chelate	500 mcg
Chromium	Chromium picolinate or chromium polynicotinate	400 mcg
Iodine	Potassium iodide	100 mcg
Magnesium	Magnesium glycinate chelate	20 mg
Manganese	Manganese glycinate chelate	3 mg
Molybdenum	Molybdenum glycinate chelate	100 mcg
Selenium	Selenomethionine	200 mcg
Zinc	Zinc glycinate chelate	15 mg
* Dosages are in international units (IU), milligrams (mg), or micrograms (mcg).		

Magnesium: 400–800 milligrams a day

Magnesium, the fourth most abundant mineral in your body, is important for more than three hundred enzymatic reactions, many of which

affect your heart. Researchers estimate that about 75 percent of us are deficient in magnesium. And a deficiency in this vital nutrient can adversely affect numerous heart conditions.

Among its benefits, magnesium helps you relax. Think about one of the most relaxing things you can do: soaking in an Epsom salt bath. When you soak in Epsom salts, you're delivering a large dose of magnesium to your body, absorbed right through your skin. And if you've ever gotten a vitamin drip from an integrative physician, you already know that there's nothing like magnesium for making you sleep like a baby.

Magnesium is a cofactor in manufacturing adenosine triphosphate (ATP), the cellular energy molecule. One study linked magnesium deficiencies to ischemic heart disease, and countless others found a connection between low levels of magnesium and poor cardiovascular health.

Magnesium also helps widen and relax blood vessels. Relaxing your arteries lets your heart pump blood more easily, thereby reducing blood pressure. Studies show that people who consume more magnesium tend to have lower blood pressure. And magnesium also helps lower blood sugar.

Taking magnesium is associated with numerous benefits, such as

- Better sleep
- Decreased muscle cramps
- Better blood pressure control
- Better blood sugar control
- Decreased constipation
- Decreased migraine headaches
- Decreased cardiac heart arrhythmias and as a result decreased risk for sudden cardiac death

Here are some examples of foods rich in magnesium (and also perfect Smart Fat Solution foods).

MAGNESIUM CONTENT IN FOOD		
	SERVING SIZE	MAGNESIUM CONTENT in mg
Nuts and seeds		
Roasted pumpkin seeds	1 oz	151
Quinoa (dry, uncooked)	¼ cup	89
Almonds	1 oz	78
Brazil nuts	1 oz	107
Cashews	1 oz	74
Beans and legumes		
Canned white beans	½ cup	67
Soybeans (edamame), cooked	½ cup	74
Black beans, cooked	½ cup	60
Peanuts	1 oz	50
Fish (cooked)		
Halibut	4 oz	120
Chinook salmon	4 oz	138
Leafy green vegetables		
Frozen spinach	½ cup	81
Swiss chard	1 cup	76
Artichoke hearts	½ cup	50

Smart Magnesium Supplementation

Magnesium is an effective way to treat constipation, if you use the right form (magnesium citrate). You'll want to avoid magnesium oxide forms of this supplement, which can produce the opposite of constipation—frequent unwanted trips to the bathroom. For best absorption, choose magnesium chelate, malate, or glycinate, though you'll likely find these in combination.

You'll often see calcium and magnesium combined, sometimes with other nutrients, in what are sold as "bone" formulas. Just remember that magnesium and calcium have a slightly complicated relationship, as calcium blocks magnesium absorption; they are best taken in a ratio of 2:1 (calcium to magnesium).

THE CALCIUM CONTROVERSY

For decades, it was a nutrition truism: Everyone should take calcium supplements to build strong bones—especially women. Now, we're not so sure.

In one study, researchers with the National Cancer Institute and several other research facilities looked at data from 388,000 men, fifty to seventy-one years of age, in six states and two big metropolitan areas.[†] The participants were followed for twelve years. Compared with men who didn't use supplements, men who consumed more than 1,000 milligrams a day of calcium from supplements had a significantly increased risk of death from heart disease by the end of the study. The problem was that the researchers didn't calculate how much calcium the men consumed in their diets, nor whether they were getting enough magnesium to balance the additional calcium.

This was just an observational study, not a clinical one, but it adds to a growing concern among many health professionals that when it comes to calcium supplements, we may have been overdoing it.

The fact is that we need calcium, especially for bone health. It's also an important ally in fighting weight gain. If you don't get at least 600–800 milligrams of calcium per day, you may notice weight gain. Menopausal women are particularly at risk.

But it's possible to get too much. Though the RDA for calcium is 1,000 milligrams a day for people nineteen to fifty years of age, that amount refers to *total calcium from diet and supplements together.* Emerging evidence indicates that many people have been under the impression that they should *supplement* with at least 1,000 milligrams a day and didn't consider the diet part of calcium intake. For example, in one study, published in the *Journal of the American Medical Association,* women who had a daily dietary intake of calcium greater than 1,400 milligrams and also took supplements had a higher cardiovascular risk than women who had the same dietary calcium and didn't take supplements.

[†] Kuehn BM. "High calcium intake linked to heart disease, death." *JAMA.* 2013; 309(10): 972.

This doesn't mean that we think you should never take calcium supplements, though we do think you need to take them in correct proportion to magnesium, ideally 2:1. But we do think you should get most, if not all, of your calcium from food sources, which does not seem to be a problem for either sex.

Only if you do not meet your calcium needs through diet should you turn to supplements to fill in the gap. Remember, the recommendations are for *total* calcium intake, not just calcium supplement intake!

Here are some good calcium food sources to help you reach 800 to 1,000 milligrams daily calcium in your diet.[†]

- Calcium-fortified almond milk, 500 milligrams per cup
- Calcium-fortified soy and coconut milk, 300 milligrams per cup
- Cow's milk (any fat content), 300 milligrams per cup
- Plain regular yogurt, 400 milligrams per cup
- Plain Greek-style yogurt, 300 milligrams per cup
- Cooked navy beans, 128 milligrams per cup
- Edamame, 100 milligrams per cup
- Kale and other cooked greens, 125 milligrams per cup
- Almonds, 75 milligrams per ounce

Add up your calcium intake for a typical day. If you are getting less than 800–1,000 milligrams daily, add a supplement so your combined diet plus supplement reaches this range. If you do supplement, avoid calcium carbonate, which you'll encounter widely as it is the cheapest form of calcium. It is sometimes contaminated with lead, and it can cause gastrointestinal problems, including constipation, particularly if it's not taken with food; also, its absorption rates are poor. Instead, choose protein-bound calcium or a calcium chelate (calcium malate chelate or calcium glycinate chelate) for the best absorption. Calcium citrate is also an option, but the absorption is not as good as protein-bound or chelate forms.

[†] We don't include hard cheese, though 1 ounce provides 100 milligrams of calcium. This is a small quantity, and because hard (organic) cheese is a neutral fat, we don't think of it as a major source of calcium since you probably will not have it more than once a day if you're following our recommendations.

Vitamin K: 250–1,000 micrograms daily

Vitamin K is essential for clotting, bone health, and preventing calcification of your arteries. Most Americans don't meet even the minimal intake guidelines for vitamin K.

Vitamin K was first identified to be essential for normal blood clotting (the "K" comes from the German word for coagulation, *Koagulieren*). Without the ability of your blood to clot, you might bleed to death from a minor cut. Over time, we've come to realize that vitamin K is also essential for bone and artery health. Without the vitamin, bones lose calcium and arteries become stiff and hard because they can't get rid of calcium from their walls.

There are two forms of vitamin K: K1 and K2. Vitamin K2 is more potent; it helps reduce calcification in the arteries and keeps calcium in the bones, where it belongs. But unless you consume big quantities of fermented soy products (such as the Japanese food natto), you won't find much in food. Vitamin K1 is easy to get from food, and most green leafy vegetables are loaded with it. A few supplements already have vitamins K1 and K2, including some of the brands we recommend, but the majority of multivitamins don't provide nearly enough for your long-term health.

How much vitamin K1 do you need for clotting? The *minimum* RDA for proper clotting is around 100 micrograms per day, but we're not interested in "minimum wage" nutrition.

Here are some great food sources of vitamin K1 that healthfully exceed that minimum:

- Cooked kale or collard greens (1 cup provides 1,000 micrograms vitamin K1)
- Cooked spinach or beets (1 cup, 700–900 micrograms)
- Broccoli or Brussels sprouts (1 cup, 220 micrograms)
- Cooked cabbage or asparagus (1 cup, about 150 micrograms)
- Onions (½ cup, 110 micrograms)

Smart Vitamin K Supplementation

If you take vitamin D and calcium, you'll absorb more calcium, but if you have low vitamin K levels, the calcium will be deposited in your arteries instead of your bones. Not good. Make sure you meet your vitamin K needs if you are taking vitamin D and/or calcium supplements. If you don't get enough vitamin K from food, then make sure you add a vitamin K supplement. Many vitamin K supplements combine a mixture of vitamins K1 and K2. If you take a supplement, aim for a total of at least 500 micrograms, with 300 micrograms as vitamin K1 and 200 micrograms as vitamin K2. Many clinicians are now recommending 1,000 mcg each of vitamins K1 and K2, a mix that's easy to find from some of the better supplement companies.

Omega-3s (Fish Oil): 1–2 grams a day

People have always lived along oceans, lakes, and rivers and have depended upon a diet rich in seafood for more than one hundred thousand years. Our health depends upon key nutrients from seafood, starting with the fats they provide—those famous long-chain omega-3 fats.

Long-chain omega-3 fatty acids, commonly called fish oil, develop in cold-water plankton and seaweed. These are consumed by shrimp, and then by bigger and bigger fish, moving on up the food chain with increasingly higher concentrations of these essential fats winding up in bigger cold-water fish like salmon.

Fish oil in our diets affects our heart in several ways. It decreases the risk for having a heart attack and stroke, improves insulin sensitivity, and decreases the risk of cardiac sudden death.

Some research has shown that fish oil supplements reduced triglyceride levels by up to 40 percent. The U.S. Agency for Healthcare Research and Quality analyzed 123 studies on omega-3 fatty acids and concluded that "omega-3 fatty acids demonstrated a consistently large, significant effect on triglycerides—a net decrease of 10 to 33 percent." The effect is most pronounced in people who have high triglycerides to begin with. Even the American Heart Association recommends 1 gram daily for most people, and for people who need to lower their triglyceride levels, up to 2 to 4 grams of the two omega-3 fats found in fish oil (EPA and DHA).

Omega-3s also lower inflammation. We consider inflammation to be one of the major promoters of heart disease, and as you know by now, inflammation is linked to diseases ranging from obesity to diabetes to cancer. Omega-3s—especially EPA and DHA—are among the most anti-inflammatory molecules ever discovered; our bodies make our own anti-inflammatory compounds called *eicosanoids* out of omega-3s, so it's vitally important to get enough of them.

In Britain, heart attack survivors are now prescribed fish oil supplements for life in keeping with the guidelines of the British National Institute for Health and Care Excellence. Many physicians also consider supplementation with omega-3 fatty acids an important part of nutritional treatment for diabetes and Metabolic Syndrome, both of which significantly increase the risk for heart disease.

Sixty percent of your brain (by weight) is made up of fat, and 25 percent of that fat is DHA. No wonder your grandmother called fish "brain food." And studies show that taking fish oil does indeed improve brain function. Low levels of omega-3 are also associated with higher rates of depression and anxiety. And epidemiological studies suggest that taking fish oil helps prevent memory loss.

Smart Omega-3 Supplementation

The two omega-3 fatty acids found in fish—EPA and DHA—are the most studied of the omega-3s and the ones that have the most demonstrated benefits. Read supplement labels and look at the amount of EPA and DHA, since that's the only part of fish oil you really need to care about. If a "big box" store sells capsules of "1,000 milligrams fish oil," don't be fooled—you need to see how much of that 1,000 milligrams is actually EPA and DHA (it will tell you on the nutrition facts label).

Remember to figure your dose on the basis of the amount of EPA and DHA, not the total amount of fish oil. If a 1,000-milligram capsule of fish oil contains 300 milligrams EPA and 200 milligrams DHA, then that capsule counts as 500 milligrams. We recommend that you get between 1,000 and 2,000 milligrams of combined EPA and DHA per day.

Some plant foods—like flax and chia—contain an omega-3, but it's a medium-chain omega-3, as opposed to the long-chain omega-3s that are found in fish. Most of the proven benefits from long-chain omega-3 fats come from marine sources, not plant sources of omega-3. The omega-3 found in flaxseed oil is called *alpha linoleic acid* (ALA). It can convert to EPA and DHA in the body, but the conversion is inefficient and only a small percentage—probably only 5 percent—winds up as EPA and DHA. However, flaxseeds have many other health benefits beyond their omega-3 content; we both recommend eating ground flaxseeds.

If you're a vegetarian, you could eat a seaweed salad several days per week or take a seaweed supplement with DHA as an effective way to benefit from omega-3 fats.[†]

Vitamin D: 2,000–3,000 IU

Vitamin D is a superstar—one of the most important supplements you can take. Vitamin D is nothing less than

- A cancer fighter
- A vital component of sex hormones
- A major player in bone strength
- A disease preventer—populations that don't get enough vitamin D through sunlight are at greater risk for developing multiple sclerosis, heart disease, and Alzheimer's
- A physical performance booster (especially in older people)

[†] One of the many wonderful things that fish oil does is thin the blood. This is normally good, but if you're taking blood-thinning medication such as warfarin (Coumadin), or have any medical condition that involves blood clotting or bleeding, be sure to discuss with your doctor any dose of fish oil more than 2 grams, as it can increase the risk for bleeding.

Even weight loss is positively affected by vitamin D. In one study, researchers measured blood levels of vitamin D in thirty-eight obese individuals before and after an eleven-week diet that contained about 750 fewer calories per day than the participants needed to maintain their weight. The low-calorie diet alone should have caused weight loss. But the researchers found that for each 1 nanogram-per-milliliter increase in blood levels of vitamin D, participants lost an additional half-pound of weight, suggesting that vitamin D might have an effect on fat metabolism. Our recent study from the database at the Masley Optimal Health Center, presented at the American College of Nutrition meeting in 2015, showed that overweight patients lost more weight if they increased their vitamin D intake.

This is not the first time that vitamin D has been linked to weight-related issues. Diabetes, for example, has long been shown to be significantly more prevalent in people with low blood levels of vitamin D. And one study showed that supplementing with vitamin D improved insulin sensitivity, a measure of how well your body metabolizes carbohydrates. (Insulin-*resistant* people are much more likely to have problems with blood sugar and weight.)

Depending upon your size and health, our recommended daily dosage of vitamin D is 2,000 to 3,000 IU, although some people with limited absorption may need 5,000 IU every day. Multivitamins typically do not have the optimal dose of vitamin D, so an additional vitamin D supplement is often a necessity.

Fortunately, there's an easy way to monitor your vitamin D levels. A simple blood test, known as the 25-hydroxy vitamin D test, will tell you precisely what your levels are. Most experts recommend that your levels be around 50 nanograms per milliliter, though some experts suggest that 40–70 nanograms per milliliter is the optimal range. Though experts disagree about what blood level is potentially toxic, we think you should keep yours to less than 70, just to be safe. Studies have shown that up to 10,000 IU a day for five months—way more than we're recommending—produces no toxicity, but that is only a short-term, not a long-term treatment plan.

Smart Vitamin D Supplementation

We strongly recommend choosing a vitamin D3 supplement. Supplemental vitamin D is available in two forms: D2 (ergocalciferol), a purely vegetarian form made from radiated yeast, and D3 (cholecalciferol), a form produced from sheep wool. Though a couple of studies have concluded that the two forms are equally valuable, most experts recommend vitamin D3 as the more potent and absorbable form, and we agree with this recommendation. One 2011 study published in the *Journal of Clinical Endocrinology and Metabolism* found that D3 supplements were 87 percent more potent in raising vitamin D levels in the blood compared with vitamin D2 supplements of the same dose. So if you choose vitamin D2, you likely have to take four to five times the dosages we recommend, and as your achieved levels vary greatly, it's even more important to check your blood levels.

Probiotics

Probiotics support the healthy bacteria living in our intestines. We have more bacteria in our guts than we have cells in our bodies, and we couldn't survive without these healthy friends. Healthy gut bacteria fight off "bad" bacteria, they lower inflammation, they metabolize drugs and hormones, they help us lose weight, they protect our hearts and brains, and they help us absorb nutrients. In short, they are essential to life.

Ideally, you want to have more "good" bacteria in your gut than "bad." When this equation is out of balance, everything from nutrient absorption, digestion, and assimilation to immune function and even weight gain is affected.

Healthy gut bacteria require fiber for their survival. With the average fiber-deficient Standard American Diet, billions of healthy bacteria starve to death. Take a course of antibiotics, and you slaughter billions more. Meanwhile, with the good bacteria significantly depleted, the bad bacteria, like weeds in a garden, can run amok. The internal ecology of your gut's garden has been destroyed. You can rebuild this inner garden by taking probiotic supplements, or eating probiotic-rich food, such as yogurt with live bacteria and other fermented foods like sauerkraut. (A yogurt that claims "live and active yogurt cultures" on the label is required to have at least five billion healthy bacteria per serving.) Typically, you'd have to ingest five to ten billion bacteria daily for several months to help restore a depleted intestinal tract. Some supplements provide thirty to sixty billion bacteria per pill to help you restore the balance more quickly.

In Steven's medical clinic, if you are prescribed an antibiotic to help fight disease, such as pneumonia, then you would take a probiotic supplement along with the antibiotic for a minimum of thirty days. Still, you'd also need to eat the ten servings of fiber (30 grams) that we suggest daily to maintain those new bacteria—otherwise, they'll just starve to death.

If you have been fiber-deprived, then we recommend you take a probiotic supplement with at least five to ten billion bacteria for at least two months to restore your gut's health. In the long term, eat probiotic-rich food and keep enjoying those ten servings of fiber every day.

EGCG (Green Tea Extract): 250–500 milligrams

We're huge fans of tea both for its health properties and as an energy drink in general. And while all tea is great, with antioxidant and anti-inflammatory benefits, one particular compound in green tea, called epigallocatechin gallate (EGCG), has been isolated and is available as a supplement. If you're not regularly drinking at least four cups of tea a day, EGCG is a supplement you should consider.

EGCG is a member of a family of substances found in tea called *catechins,* which are in turn a member of a larger class of plant chemicals called *polyphenols.* Polyphenols are thought to be responsible for a large part of the health benefits of tea, but EGCG in particular is of special interest. It sparks heat production in the body, or *thermo-genesis* (*thermo* means "heat," and *genesis* means "making new"). You may know the process of thermogenesis by its more common term: fat burning. And sure enough, EGCG has been found to be of great interest to people who are trying to manage their weight.

In a 2010 study published in the *Journal of the American College of Nutrition,* researchers randomly assigned thirty-five obese subjects with metabolic syndrome to one of three study conditions. The control group drank four cups of water a day; the second group drank four cups of green tea a day; and the third drank two cups of green tea extract supplements of EGCG plus four cups of water a day. (Both the tea-only and the supplement-plus-water group received the same amount of EGCG per day, whether it came from the tea or the supplement.) The researchers found that both the group drinking the green tea and the group taking the EGCG supplements experienced a significant decrease in body weight and body mass index. The controls saw no such decrease.

This is hardly the first time that green tea or green tea supplements have been shown to have a positive effect on various health risk factors, nor is it the first time they've been shown to have a positive effect on fat loss and body weight. A 2009 study found that a blend of tea polyphenols derived from green tea improved both lipid (fat) and glucose (sugar) metabolism in animals. The tea supplement also enhanced insulin sensitivity and balanced the metabolic rate of fat burning with the metabolic rate of fat deposit (meaning that nothing extra was stored as fat!).

Green Tea Helps Burn Calories

Green tea consumption leads to a significant increase in calorie burning, a decrease in body weight, and a decrease in waist circumference, all while producing no real change in heart rate or blood pressure. Researchers suspect that one of the ways it accomplishes this is by possibly prolonging the effects of norepinephrine, one of the stimulating chemicals in the body. Traditional Chinese medicine has long recommended green tea as a general tonic for energy and for all sorts of ailments and conditions, including headaches, body aches and pains, digestion, depression, immune enhancement, and detoxification.

This makes sense. In a 1999 study published in the *American Journal of Clinical Nutrition*, researchers measured energy expenditure (calories burned) in ten healthy young men who were randomly given either a standard green tea extract (375 milligrams of catechins and 150 milligrams of caffeine), 150 milligrams of caffeine by itself, or an inert placebo. Believe it or not, the caffeine was no better than the placebo at speeding up metabolism, but the men receiving the green tea extract burned an average of 78 calories a day more. A 2005 study published in the *British Journal of Nutrition* found that the increased calorie burn was a little higher—about 178 calories a day from a combination of 200 milligrams of caffeine and any dose of EGCG tested, from 90 to 400 milligrams.

Although that amount of calories per day isn't enormous, it's still significant, and those calories do add up. It's hard to argue that EGCG isn't a great addition to a supplement program when you consider all the other health benefits besides "metabolism boosting": the fact that studies show zero negative effects (for example, no increase in heart rate), and the fact that green tea tends to stimulate both calorie burning and fat burning.

Nutritionist Shari Lieberman, in her book *Dare to Lose,* pointed out that green tea stimulates the metabolism to a far greater degree than a comparable amount of caffeine alone. "It appears that . . . EGCG stimulates the production of noradrenaline, which in turns revs up your metabolism," Lieberman wrote. "Studies have shown that using green tea even without restricting food (dieting) causes weight loss—using it with a weight-loss eating plan should give you excellent results."

Beyond weight loss, green tea has other benefits. Tea drinkers have a lower risk of heart attack and stroke, less gum disease, and better bone density and lower fracture rates. We highly encourage you to enjoy three to four cups of green tea daily, and if you need help with weight loss and don't like green tea, then consider an EGCG supplement.

Although we have focused on EGCG, there are lots of benefits to drinking tea, so enjoy it as long as it isn't sweetened. Green tea, however, has the highest concentration of EGCG.

Curcumin: 500 milligrams daily (dosing varies from 400 to 1,000 milligrams)

Curcumin is the name given to a collection of compounds called *curcuminoids,* which are the active anti-inflammatory compound found in the super-spice turmeric. Curcumin is not only a powerful anti-inflammatory, it also provides antioxidant, antithrombotic, and cardiovascular protective benefits. Among its heart duties, curcumin reduces oxidized LDL cholesterol.

Because of these powerful properties, curcumin is used to decrease arthritis symptoms by lowering joint inflammation. As we mentioned in Chapter 2, it has been used in cancer prevention and treatment studies, and researchers are using it to decrease memory loss. One 2012 study published in the *British Journal of Pharmacology* found that curcumin could preserve cardiac function after heart attack.

We think it's got a lot more than just "potential"—both of us take it every day.

Smart Curcumin Tips

Turmeric spice is not well absorbed, and you're unlikely to get enough curcumin from food even if you sprinkle turmeric on everything you eat. To get 500 milligrams of curcumin daily, you'd need to ingest about three heaping tablespoons of turmeric every day. So supplements are the way to go. Yet, curcumin is poorly absorbed, and

VITAMIN C, WHERE ARE YOU?

You may notice that we do not include vitamin C—one of the most important antioxidants in the world—in our list of additional supplements. This is not because we don't think it's important. We do.

A large study published in 2011 found that the lower the amount of vitamin C in the blood, the higher the risk of heart failure. Oxidative damage is a huge contributor to every major disease, and vitamin C is one of the most powerful antioxidants available, so getting plenty of vitamin C through food and supplements is a high priority.

We think you should be getting (at least) 1,000 milligrams of vitamin C a day from diet and supplements. (Jonny would go a bit higher, Steven would go a bit lower, but we both agree that 1,000 milligrams makes sense.) We've made the assumption that there's 250 milligrams in your multivitamin (which may not always be true) and that you would be getting at least 750 milligrams a day of vitamin C from food by following the Smart Fat Solution eating recommendations.

But if your vitamin C intake falls short of 1,000 milligrams a day through diet and a multivitamin, we do recommend an additional vitamin C supplement.

cheap brands have been reported to be contaminated with heavy metals, making a high-quality curcumin product essential if you wish to benefit from taking curcumin as a supplement. Look for the quality brands we recommended early in this chapter.

Coenzyme Q10: 60-200 milligrams

Coenzyme Q10 (or CoQ10) is a vitally important nutrient that recharges the energy-production furnaces in the cells (the mitochondria). It's one of the greatest nutrients for energy, and since the heart cells produce more energy than any other organ, CoQ10 and the heart are a natural fit. Indeed, CoQ10 has been approved as a drug to treat congestive heart failure in Japan since 1974—it's that effective at helping the heart produce energy.

Nearly every cell in your body makes CoQ10, but as we age we produce substantially less of it. And don't think you're going to make up the difference with food—CoQ10 is found in only small quantities in food, mainly in organ meats (heart, liver, and kidney). Other foods that have it, such as sardines and beef, contain tiny amounts—you'd need a ton of these foods to get even 30 milligrams a day, the absolute minimum dose for healthy folks needing general protection.

CoQ10 is required in order for your body to manufacture ATP (adenosine triphosphate), the "gasoline" that makes every cell run and every muscle move. ATP becomes especially crucial for heart health since your heart is your most metabolically active tissue; it demands a constant supply of these energy molecules.

CoQ10 can also reduce blood pressure. A meta-analysis published in 2007 in the *Journal of Human Hypertension* reviewed twelve different clinical trials and found that people receiving CoQ10 supplementation had significant reductions in blood pressure compared with control subjects who didn't receive supplementation. No wonder several studies have demonstrated a strong correlation between the severity of heart disease and CoQ10 deficiency.

Your heart actually contains the greatest concentration of CoQ10 in the body. Simply put, your heart *loves* CoQ10.

Smart Coenzyme Q10 Supplementation

Recently, there's been quite a controversy in the nutrition community over what form of CoQ10 is best to take: ubiquinone or ubiquinol. For years, manufacturers offered CoQ10 as ubiquinone. This is still what's most frequently found in CoQ10 supplements, and it's the form that the bulk of the research on CoQ10 has investigated. Supplement companies now offer CoQ10 as ubiquinol, and many believe that this form, which is the active form of CoQ10 in the body, is a more potent, better absorbed form. The jury is still out on whether one form is better than the other. We think you can't go wrong with either one, though people who have trouble absorbing this nutrient may do better with the (more expensive) ubiquinol.

One group of people who definitely need CoQ10 supplements are those taking statin drugs, the main class of medication used to reduce cholesterol. Statin drugs significantly deplete CoQ10, lowering levels about 20 percent, so if you're taking a statin, it's very important to supplement with this nutrient. If you're not on a statin, we recommend 60–100 milligrams a day from a high-quality product that has excellent absorption. At some point you can ask your physician to check your CoQ10 level to confirm that you are adequately dosed. A CoQ10 blood level between 1.5 to 2.5 is optimal.

Absorption is a major consideration with CoQ10. Tablet forms typically have only a 1 percent absorption rate, which is poor. Oil-based capsules should have at least a 4 percent absorption rate. Some high-quality brands, like Thorne and Designs for Health, have published absorption rates that exceed 8 percent. If you're taking CoQ10, don't try saving money by buying an inexpensive form that doesn't get into your bloodstream. In this case, paying more for better quality may actually save you money.

Resveratrol: 100–250 milligrams (of trans-resveratrol)

Resveratrol—an anti-aging nutrient found primarily in red wine and the skins of dark grapes—protects your arteries against blood clots, improves their elasticity, and reduces blood pressure and oxidized LDL cholesterol. A powerful antioxidant and anti-inflammatory compound, resveratrol inhibits several inflammatory enzymes. Recent research shows that it also helps manage blood sugar and has a positive effect on insulin resistance in diabetics. Resveratrol also stops certain molecules from sticking to artery walls, where they hang out and create inflammation.

Resveratrol upregulates—the scientific term for "turning up the volume"—some of the longevity genes that are activated by calorie restriction. Studies have shown that decreasing your caloric intake in the long term by at least 20 percent may slow the aging process; the obvious challenge is that you feel like you are starving all the time. Resveratrol mimics some of these longevity gene activation benefits while allowing you to eat a normal, healthy diet.

Smart Resveratrol Supplementation

The active part of resveratrol is called *trans-resveratrol,* and it's this active ingredient that has the benefit. If you read the fine print on the label, most resveratrol supplements will say something like "standardized to 10 percent trans-resveratrol," which sounds great, but really this means that only 10 percent of what's in the pill is the kind of resveratrol you actually care about. So, for example, if a capsule is labeled as containing 500 milligrams resveratrol but is standardized to 10 percent trans-resveratrol, you're getting only about 50 milligrams of trans-resveratrol for every 500-milligram pill you take (10 percent of 500 milligrams is 50 milligrams).

Though the exact optimal dose of trans-resveratrol is unknown, most experts agree that 100–250 milligrams is a meaningful amount. Some companies, such as Reserveage Nutrition and Thorne Research, offer resveratrol supplements that are 100 percent trans-resveratrol, but most companies do not. Read the label.

VERY HONORABLE MENTION: CITRUS BERGAMOT

Other supplements can also be useful, and we're learning more and more about their benefits all the time. For instance, emerging research on the extract of the bergamot orange—a fruit native to Italy that is used to flavor Earl Grey tea—suggests that it can improve the symptoms of Metabolic Syndrome by lowering blood sugar and triglycerides and increasing HDL cholesterol

You personally may not need to take every one of the supplements we have explored here, but these are our recommendations, in conjunction with the Smart Fat Solution. Your health practitioner, or a nutritionist, should be able to help you customize a regimen for your unique biochemical needs. We anticipate that you will tailor our supplement recommendations to complement the nutrients you consume from food, with a daily pill count that is realistic for you and a budget you can afford. For details on balancing how many pills you take per day and quality supplement pricing, visit www.SmartFat.com. As noted, our bare minimum recommendation is that you take a high-quality multivitamin with adequate vitamin D daily, and that from a combination of food and supplements, you meet your optimal health needs for magnesium, vitamin K, and fish oil.

But remember that supplements are no more, and no less, than what they claim they are: supplements, and they are only supplemental to a healthy eating plan. They will not take the place of a healthy smart fat diet, but in many cases they can add a lot of value.

Jonny's mentor, the nutritionist Robert Crayhon, once said about supplements: "There are two common mistakes when it comes to nutritional supplements: thinking they do nothing, or thinking they do everything."

We couldn't agree more.

CHAPTER 9

Smart Living

THE SMART FAT SOLUTION is a safe, scientifically sound, effective way to lose weight, restore your health, and reclaim your energy. But it's *not* the whole story.

This statement may have you thinking, "Here comes the chapter where they pay lip service to all the lifestyle stuff." Trust us—as you've trusted us so far—it's anything but lip service. What you do *beyond food* is vitally important to your quality of life.

Smart fat eating virtually guarantees that you'll be putting top-grade fuel in your personal energy tank. That one change alone will have a dramatic, immediate, and positive effect on everything from your weight to your energy level. But that's just the beginning.

You see, your body is like your car: No matter how good the gas you put in the tank is, it's not the only thing you need to get top performance out of your engine. It needs spark plugs. It needs oil changes. It needs regular maintenance. Only then will the engine perform the way it's really capable of performing.

Which brings us to this chapter.

Smart Fat eating is only the first part of a five-part program. We

have spent the bulk of this book on food—the gas for your engine—
because eating the smart fat way will have the quickest and most dramatic effects on your overall well-being, not to mention your weight.
But food is only part one. Now we're going to cover the other four parts:
exercise, stress reduction, sleep, and relationships.

Please don't skip this chapter. By spending time on each of the four
areas covered here, you will be virtually guaranteed to turbo-charge
your results, increase your performance and stamina, feel lighter,
freer . . . and happier!

After all, people don't read a book like this if they don't believe it
can help them have a better life. And one of the keys to a better life is
managing one of the only metrics you can measure every single day:
your own energy. When you have boundless energy, you tend to have
boundless enthusiasm. You begin to be more optimistic. You see the
bright side of things, and you act accordingly, assuming that what you
do can actually make a difference. People notice you in a different way.
You'll seem—and perhaps even look—lighter.

But to get all of these benefits from the Smart Fat Solution—
benefits we know can be yours—you'll have to do a few other things
besides eat right.

Smart Exercise

Let's not mince words. Exercise is the single most potent anti-aging
"drug" ever invented. Daily moderate exercise—and we define what
we mean by that below—reduces your risk of developing diabetes,
obesity, depression, cancer, and heart disease. It also may fight off the
baby boomer's greatest fear: loss of mind. (Few things generate more
fear among baby boomers than Alzheimer's disease.)

Give Your Brain a Boost

For a long time we've known that exercise strengthens the heart
and improves cardiovascular health. Makes sense, doesn't it? The

heart is a muscle, and if you exercise it, it will get stronger, just like the biceps or the quadriceps. And the job of the heart—one of them, anyway—is to pump oxygen and nutrients to all the cells, organs, and tissues in the body so that they can function optimally.

One of those organs that need oxygen and nutrients is the brain. So it stands to reason that if you want to keep your brain healthy, vibrant, and functioning, you want to continue to supply it with everything it needs to keep things running efficiently. Coincidentally, the best way to do this is to keep your heart pumping! And not surprisingly, a lot of research has shown that exercise does in fact improve brain function. Research published from the Masley Optimal Health Center confirms that greater fitness improves executive function and brain performance.

Until recently, no one looked at whether exercise had an effect on the anatomy of the brain. Now it seems that actual physical changes in the brain—all of them positive—occur as a result of aerobic exercise. In fact, it's now possible to say with scientific certainty that aerobic exercise makes your brain bigger!

Here's what happened. Dr. Arthur Kramer and his colleagues at the University of Illinois took a group of sixty older people who were healthy but sedentary and looked at their brains using magnetic resonance imaging (MRI). Then he divided them into two groups. Half of them began a gentle, easy aerobics program, and the other half began a "toning and stretching" program.

The aerobics program started off slowly, with about fifteen minutes a day of walking. After about two months, the subjects were up to forty-five to sixty minutes of walking three days a week. (Most covered a few miles during that time frame, meaning they were walking at about four miles per hour.) The subjects kept this up for six months.

Then everyone had another MRI done, and Kramer and his team looked at the grey and white matter in the subjects' brains. "Grey matter," you may recall from science class, is composed of the actual neurons of the brain—the "computational units." "White matter," on the other hand, is made up of the axons, or interconnections between the neurons. The researchers wanted to see whether the functional improvement in the brain that had been observed in so much research on exercise and the brain was accompanied by any physical changes.

And it was. Amazingly, the subjects in the aerobics group showed an increase in volume in both the grey matter *and* the white matter of their brains.

The take-away from this is a pretty clear, especially for those of us interested in keeping our brains healthy and operational well into our eighties and beyond: Exercise! And the beautiful part is that it doesn't take much exercise to do this. According to Kramer, the amount of exercise needed for the brain-building effect is pretty moderate— forty-five to sixty minutes of walking three times a week. It's a wonderful confirmation of why moderate exercise is such an important part of your nutrition program.

Steven has published studies from his own clinic showing that the combination of a smart fat diet and exercise—thirty to sixty minutes, five times a week—increases brain speed and executive performance by a whopping 30 percent—a pretty nice improvement in mental sharpness!

What Exercise Should I Do?

There are a lot of ways to get in shape; people are passionate about yoga, aerobics, weight training, circuit training, interval training, burst training, Pilates, kick boxing, step classes, and Crossfit, to name just a few. In fact, any one of these can provide significant benefits. Ultimately, the best exercise program for you is the exercise program that you actually *do*.

When Jonny started his career in the early 1990s as a trainer at Equinox, the New York–based fitness club, a woman came into the gym who, according to all the trainers on staff, was the fittest specimen of humanity they had ever seen. All the trainers were eager to find out what magical combination of cardio and weights this woman did to get in such fabulous shape, since they all hoped to copy her routine and use it with their clients. Eventually, one of the trainers approached the woman. "Would you mind telling us," he asked shyly, "how you got in such astonishing shape?"

Her answer, said with a Texas drawl: "Ropin' cattle."

The point is that virtually any exercise can work as long as you *do it*. Our "prescription" for exercise, therefore, is going to be more general and philosophical than specific. There are tons of books, videos, and programs that will tell you exactly what exercises to do and in what order; they can take you through workouts ranging from easy to moderate to insane.

But rather than give you a specific routine, we give you a few general guidelines, which come down to two things: *work your heart* and *work your muscles.* If you make a commitment to be active every day, you'll soon find yourself gravitating to some forms of exercise more than others, and eventually you'll wind up with a routine that fits your lifestyle. You may even find that you stop thinking of exercise as "exercise"—it will instead be a part of your life.

Get Moving with Walking

Walking is probably the least controversial and most studied form of exercise, the one action that has copious proven benefits with just about no downside. At the very least, try to take a walk three to five days a week. It requires no investment, no special equipment, no gym, no nothing.

A significant amount of emerging research in the field of exercise argues for the benefit of short, intense workouts (interval training). This kind of workout—also known as high-intensity interval training (HIIT) or burst training—is based on the notion that you get more out of a workout if you alternate periods of intense effort with periods of "active rest."

So, for example, if you were jogging or walking briskly on a treadmill at a comfortable speed of, say, 4, interval training would have you push it for thirty to sixty seconds to a speed of 6 and then come back down to 3 for a minute of "recovery" (i.e., active rest). A period of high intensity (treadmill speed of 6) alternating with a period of active rest (treadmill speed of 3) would constitute one "set," and you can do up to ten sets like this in one workout—all in less than thirty minutes. Ten minutes on a treadmill alternating between "high intensity" and "low intensity" can be as effective as thirty minutes at a slow, even (and nonchallenging) pace. With this kind of training, you work out smarter, not necessarily harder. You accomplish just as much—if not more—and in less time.

You can introduce interval training into your daily walk easily, even if you're just beginning to exercise or just starting up again after a long layoff. When you're doing your walk at your normal pace, try speeding it up for thirty seconds. Then slow down while you catch your breath, and then, after a bit, repeat the sequence. You'll be pushing your fitness envelope in no time.

Use It or Lose It: Weight Training

In addition to getting moving, you'll need to do something to preserve your muscles, and this generally means *training with weights*. If you don't do some form of strength training (weights), expect to lose about 1 pound of muscle every year. Remember that muscle not only looks good, it's also the place where you burn most of your calories. So when you lose muscle, you're actually losing some of your body's calorie-burning furnaces, which means you're slowing down your metabolism. Since there are fewer places to burn calories, the calories you're eating are more easily stored as fat, and your body shape changes dramatically even if your weight stays stable. Muscle is your best friend in the battle of the bulge. When talking about muscle, the old adage is true: "Use it or lose it." If you want to get (or stay) lean, you'd better use it.

We suggest you train with weights at least twice a week. It doesn't have to be a long, drawn-out, exhausting workout. We both do our entire weight workout in fewer than thirty minutes. Jonny does a circuit of exercises, one for each major body part—chest, back, shoulders, biceps, triceps, legs, and abs—and then rests for a minute and repeats the circuit twice more. He's in and out of the gym in about twenty-five minutes. Steven does two days of upper-body strength training and two days of trunk and lower-body strength training, alternating upper-body days with lower-body days, in workouts that last about fifteen to twenty minutes. The point here is that there are lots of ways to accomplish the same goal.

Yes, This Is Exercise, Too: The Fun Stuff

Finally, there's the fun stuff—*the stuff that doesn't feel like exercise but is.* Taking a hike. Walking the dogs. Gardening. Playing tennis. (Interesting factoid: Tennis players have the lowest resting heart rates of any athletes. And resting heart rate is a terrific metric for general fitness. If your resting heart rate is low [under sixty beats per minute]—as it is with world-class athletes—it means your heart doesn't have to work so hard!) Find something you like to do, and then *do it.*

For inspiration, it's worth paying attention to the findings of the National Weight Control Registry, which has been tracking the activities of people who are winners at the weight-loss game. It's the largest prospective investigation of long-term successful weight-loss maintenance ever done. The registry has been tracking more than ten thousand individuals who have maintained at least thirty pounds of weight loss for one year or longer, though the average member has lost an astonishing sixty pounds and has kept it off for five years!

Several behavior patterns have emerged from the findings, but one of them is of particular interest: A full 90 percent of the participants exercise about one hour a day. Women in the registry report expending an average of 2,545 calories a week in physical activity, and men report an average of 3,293 calories a week. The most common activity is walking, reported by 76 percent of the participants. An additional 20 percent lift weights, 20 percent cycle, and 18 percent do aerobics.

Exercise Recommendations

So for those of you who want to lose weight and keep it off, what are our *minimal* recommendations? And for those who are more ambitious, what are our *optimal* recommendations?

Minimally, we believe that the combination of walking, or another form of aerobic exercise, at least three to four times a week plus twice-weekly weight training is the best basic template from which to build a personal activity program. If you combine this basic level of exercise with the Smart Fat Solution eating plan, you'll be virtually assured of getting great results—and we're pretty sure you'll like what you see in the mirror.

Our optimal recommendations are the following:

1. Aerobic training five to six days per week with some combination of the following:

   —High-intensity interval training (HIIT) at least two to three days a week

   —One to two hours of a moderate, fun activity, such as a long walk, a hike, a bicycle ride, tennis, or golf, two days a week (on non-HIIT days)

2. Strength training at least two days a week

3. Yoga, swimming, or prolonged stretching at least once a week

Our minimal recommendations will give you great results. But if you're able to follow the optimal plan, you'll look and feel even better. Remember, though, as we have said, *the best exercise program is the one you actually do,* so pick something that's realistic for you and that you're likely to stick with in the long term.

Smart Stress Reduction

Whenever Jonny talks to audiences about stress, he brings up the case of Cindy Gore.

Cindy, along with her husband Russell, lived in New Orleans. They were there in August 2005 when Hurricane Katrina struck, and their home was flooded with 9 feet of water. Russell and Cindy climbed to the attic and waited for rescue helicopters. Russell kept his arms around his wife, whispering reassuring words and telling her not to panic.

"The next thing I know," Russell told Gary Tuchman of CNN, "I was talking to her, she leaned over and she was dead."

Cindy Gore—a healthy, robust woman in her fifties—had died of stress.

This heartbreaking story illustrates something that few people fully appreciate: Stress kills. It may not kill as dramatically and quickly as it did in the case of Cindy Gore, but kill it does—slowly and insidiously. It can exacerbate (or even initiate) outbreaks of "minor" conditions like herpes, asthma, allergies, and acne, and it worsens just about every degenerative disease of aging—from cancer to diabetes to heart disease. It slows down recovery from serious illness. In the brain, it shrinks the hippocampus, an area that's intimately involved in memory and thinking. It increases the risk of cardiovascular disease. It decreases the effectiveness of the immune system. (Jonny has referred to stress as one of the "Four Horsemen of Aging," and some might argue that it is the most deadly "horseman" of them all.)

Stress is a lot more than a mere annoyance or an inconvenient fact of modern life. It's a true life-shortener and probably the single most potent enemy of health and longevity on the planet. We tell you this not to frighten you, but to make you aware that stress management is *not* a luxury. If you want the lifetime of robust good health that the Smart Fat Solution can give you, you must deal with stress in a productive way. Ignoring it isn't an option.

Stress: A Physiological History

The stress response is a multidimensional, complicated set of hormonal and biochemical responses and signals that affect virtually the entire body. Stress is most definitely *not* "all in your head"—you can actually measure blood (and saliva) levels of specific stress-related hormones (such as cortisol and didehydroepiandrosterone [DHEA]). And like many things we wish we weren't stuck with—cravings for sugar, for example—the stress response plays a critical role in our survival.

Imagine that you're resting peacefully in the African Serengeti, and all of a sudden a hungry lion charges you. What do you do? Well, obviously, you run like hell. Or you pick up the nearest weapon to fight the beast off. But even before you consciously decide what you're going to do, your body has sprung into action. A tiny area deep in the brain called the *amygdala* registers danger even before you're aware of it. The amygdala immediately sends a message to the "air-traffic controller" of hormones in your brain known as the *hypothalamus*. The hypothalamus relays a hormonal signal to the pituitary gland, which in turn sends a hormonal signal to the intended target of all this rapid-fire communication: the adrenal glands, which sit perched atop the kidneys. All of this happens faster than you can press the "send" button after you write an email.

The adrenals are responsible for sending out powerful hormones—cortisol and adrenaline—that immediately set in motion a number of important things that need to happen if you're going to escape the lion. Number one, they get your heart racing. Number two, they shut off other metabolic operations that you don't need right at the moment, such as digestion. (Why bother to digest food if you're about to *become* food?) The stress hormones are like a first gear for the body, meant to pull you out of an emergency and prepare your body to either fight or flee—which is why they're also referred to as "the fight or flight hormones."

Stress hormones are responsible for making you instantly alert, locked and loaded, ready for action. Your blood courses through your veins. Your blood pressure goes up. Your pupils dilate (so you can see where you're going when you run). Your blood sugar rises (you'll need it for energy). Your heart races. These are all good things—if you want to survive a lion or other emergency. After all, if it weren't for stress hormones, you wouldn't react any differently to a lion than you would to a Mozart piano concerto—and that wouldn't be very good for the survival of the species.

Our ancient physiology programmed us to survive life-threatening emergencies like lions and tigers and bears. And like first gear on a car, this metabolic machinery was meant to be used infrequently. The problem is that the primitive regions of our brains where all this plays out can't tell the difference between a lion and a traffic jam, or between a wild boar and a demanding boss. The near constant stress of daily life puts our physiology on perpetual alert. And when we're in a continuous state of stress, cortisol is always elevated—and this is anything but good news.

High levels of cortisol increase insulin resistance, Metabolic Syndrome, and heart disease. High levels of stress hormones like cortisol lower immunity (which is why marathoners—who put their body through enormous physical stress during an event—often get sick the week after). Cortisol also breaks down muscle and causes your body to gain weight, most especially around the middle (the dreaded belly fat that gives you an "apple shape"). And that fat around the middle happens to be the most metabolically active and dangerous fat on your body, greatly increasing the risk for all sorts of bad things (such as heart disease).

This is why stress management is not an optional "add-on" to the Smart Fat Solution. It's essential for its success.

Back in the day when Jonny was a senior trainer at Equinox Fitness Club, he had a number of female clients who were working out like crazy but seemed unable to change their body compositions. They found it incredibly hard to build tight, toned muscle and equally hard to lose belly fat, which, weirdly enough, many of them actually seemed to be *gaining*. (Of course, many of them were on low-fat diets, which would explain part of the problem—but not all of it.) Only many years later did Jonny come to understand the reason for this: stress.

Elevated levels of cortisol will break down muscle and add belly fat and will keep you from extracting every last bit of value you can get from the Smart Fat Solution. That's why it's so deeply and profoundly important that you do something every day to moderate your stress and calm down your cortisol.

This is where deep breathing, meditation, and calming exercises come in. Deep breathing, yoga, tai chi, qi gong, stretching, and relaxing all help rehabilitate the body and the damage that constantly elevated cortisol brought to it courtesy of modern life.

The beautiful part about stress reduction is that it's easy, fun, relaxing, and inexpensive. All you have to do is find something you like to do and then do it. Maybe it's reading a novel or taking a warm bubble bath or going for a walk after dinner. Sure, meditation, yoga, and other such activities are terrific, but you can let off some steam and calm your physiology with even less of an effort. *Just relax.* Take some time for yourself—and do it every day. Caretakers have a lot of trouble with this concept. They seem to be hardwired to attend to the needs of others and frequently forget about their own. If this is you, it's good to remember what they tell you on airplanes: Put on *your own* oxygen mask first, *before* you help the person next to you—even if that person is your kid.

Plenty of books are out there about how to manage stress, as well as programs to help you do it, but here's one easy thing you can do right now at home that will make a difference. Do this exercise every day and you're guaranteed to feel better and improve your health at the same time.

Stress Recommendation: Practice Deep Breathing

For ten minutes every day, do this simple, deep-breathing exercise:

1. Sit quietly in a comfortable position (or lie down on your back, palms facing upward).
2. Close your eyes.
3. Gradually relax all your muscles one by one, starting at your feet and moving up to your face.

4. Breathe in deeply through your nose and out through your mouth.

5. Concentrate only on your breathing. But don't worry if your mind wanders (it will)—just come back to noticing your breath.

As you breathe out, silently say a calming word to yourself. It can be as simple as "peace," "joy," "love," "quiet," or even "gratitude."

Smart Sleep

If you want to check in with yourself on the quality of your life, there's probably no better metric to look at than your energy level. When you have tons of energy, life is generally good. When you don't . . . well, not so much.

These days, lots of us don't have much energy. Perhaps you've noticed. We're tired. We're dragging at work. We can't wake up in the morning, and when we do drag ourselves out of bed, we're groggy. Irritability—an inevitable accompaniment to fatigue—is a constant presence. Our work suffers, our sex life suffers, our relationships suffer, our health suffers.

So what's up with that? Why are we so tired all the time?

One of the principles of science is called the *principle of parsimony,* which holds that the simplest explanation for a phenomenon is often the best one. Or, as one of Jonny's professors once said, "When you hear hoofbeats outside your window, don't start off looking for zebras." In other words, when you're looking for an explanation, begin with the obvious (in the case of the hoofbeats, look for a horse). The obvious cause for our flagging energy is right under our noses: We're not sleeping enough.

It's All About the Rhythm

Before the invention of electricity, we were much more in tune with our biological, or *circadian,* rhythms (from the Latin *circa,* "around," and *diem,* "day"). Brainwave activity, hormone production, and all sorts of other regulatory metabolic functions are deeply connected to our circadian rhythms. These same rhythms that are such an essential part of our biological makeup are actually triggered by external events, the most important of which are light and dark. Our bodies essentially come preloaded with the software for sleeping when it's dark and waking when it's light. When our sleep patterns deviate from this programming, metabolic and hormonal systems break down and all kinds of problems occur (which is one of the many reasons why shift workers are plagued with so many health issues).

Sleep affects how we work, how we relate to people, how we perform, how we make decisions, how much energy we have, and how we feel overall. The effect of sleep, or lack of it, is profound and probably influences every metric of our existence. Sleeping too little depresses our immune systems, raises our stress hormones, and, incidentally, makes us fat. (We knew that would get your attention.)

The Wake-Up Call: Weight Gain

If the connection between gaining weight and not sleeping enough comes as a surprise, consider this. Sleep greatly affects your hormones, and when it comes to weight gain, hormones basically run the show. Sleeping poorly, or not sleeping enough, throws a monkey wrench into the complex interplay of hormones that control appetite and body weight.

Research has found that short sleep duration is associated with reduced leptin (the hormone that tells your brain you're full) (see Chapter 2 for more on leptin). For a double whammy, it's also associated with increased levels of ghrelin (a hormone that signals to the brain that you're hungry), virtually compelling you to eat. With *less* of the hormone that tells you you're full, and *more* of the hormone that tells you you're hungry, it's no wonder scientists have long observed an association between short habitual sleep time and increased weight.

It gets worse.

Recent research has shown that not getting enough sleep reduces the ability of your cells to respond to insulin. You may recall the ability of the cells to "listen" to insulin—a desirable state of affairs called insulin sensitivity (see Chapter 2). This is a hallmark of healthy weight and of good health in general. Its opposite, insulin resistance, is an undesirable state of affairs that happens when the cells no longer pay attention to insulin. The cells, particularly the muscle cells, close their doors when insulin comes calling with its sugar payload. The sugar winds up going to the fat cells (and everyone knows how *that* story ends). Insulin resistance, as you learned earlier, is a hallmark of both diabetes and obesity, and a big risk factor for heart disease.

Lack of sleep makes you insulin resistant. And no matter how brilliantly you are eating, if your insulin isn't working properly—if the cells aren't listening to it—you're likely to get fat. Are you beginning to see why sleep is so essential to your success with the Smart Fat Solution?

In one study, J. L. Broussard and colleagues at the University of Chicago had seven healthy, lean young adults live in a sleep laboratory for four days on two occasions spaced about a month apart. They ate identical meals and were not allowed to eat snacks. In the first part of the study, the subjects spent 8½ hours in bed for each of the four nights in the sleep lab. For the second part of the study, they slept only 4½ hours a night, so that by the end of the second part of the study they were sleep-deprived by about fourteen hours.

After each four-day period, the researchers measured the participants' insulin response. They also collected fat cells in order to measure how those fat cells reacted to insulin after fourteen hours of sleep deprivation.

The results were not encouraging. After only four nights of sleep deprivation, the participants' overall ability to respond to insulin had decreased by 16 percent—and that's in healthy young subjects after only four nights of not sleeping enough! One can imagine the metabolic havoc wrecked upon older, less resilient adults after years of not sleeping enough. It's not a pretty picture.

Exactly what happens when we sleep, and why we need sleep in the first place, remains a bit of a mystery—even to scientists who study this stuff. And although scientists don't fully understand exactly *why* our bodies need sleep, they know that they *do*. Sleep generates hormones, such as human growth hormone, the ultimate "anti-aging" hormone that's released only during the deep stages of sleep. (Human growth hormone helps you build muscle and burn fat, while stimulating cell reproduction and regeneration.) During deep sleep your body also produces *melatonin,* a hormone that helps regulate the sleep cycle and also has some anticancer activity to boot.

While a good night's sleep has a positive effect on hormones, a lack of sleep has a negative effect. Lack of sleep is a huge stressor on the body, which causes you to release more cortisol (the stress hormone), which, as you've seen, can create belly fat, break down muscle, shrink the brain, and depress the immune system. (It can also make you overeat like crazy.)

The Architecture of Sleep (and What Happens When the Foundation Cracks)

To appreciate just how important sleep is to your health—and why extended, uninterrupted, deep, and restful sleep may be one of the most important things you can do to manage your weight and regain your health—it helps to know something about what's called *sleep architecture.* Sleep can be divided into two categories: REM (rapid eye movement) sleep and non-REM sleep.

Non-REM sleep is divided into four stages. Stage one is that period when you first move from wakefulness to drowsiness to falling asleep. (Think of nodding off late at night while watching television.) In stage two, eye movements stop, brain waves begin to slow, muscles start to relax, heart rate slows, and body temperature starts to drop. Stages three and four are together known as slow wave sleep and are characterized by brain waves known as delta waves. During slow wave sleep, your blood pressure and body temperature drop a bit more, breathing slows more, and the body becomes immobile. (This is what we call the "dead to the world" phase.)

And then there's REM sleep, the jewel in the crown, the pièce de résistance of deep, restorative sleep. This is when the cast of characters in your own personal dreamland come alive and dance. (REM sleep is the only stage when you dream). One complete sleep cycle consists of the four stages of non-REM sleep plus REM sleep and takes a total of about 90–110 minutes. Ideally, the cycle is repeated about four to six times a night.

But as we age, everything changes. It takes longer to fall asleep. The percentage of time we spend in each stage changes; we spend a little longer in stages one and two, and a little less in stages three, four, and REM sleep (meaning we spend just a little less time in deep sleep). Regardless, normal healthy adults should still spend about 25 percent of their sleep time in REM sleep—and when this is disrupted, all kinds of stuff happens, none of it good. (There's a reason why sleep deprivation is used as a torture technique.)

We've already discussed how sleep affects weight and how not sleeping enough increases stress. But sleep is also essential to memory, mood, and cognitive performance. Lack of sleep is linked to increased anger, anxiety, and sadness—all metrics for a poor quality of life. One study showed that when subjects were permitted to sleep only 4½ hours a night, they exhibited significantly more stress, mental exhaustion, and anger.

Sleep also affects immunity. In one clever study, researchers gave flu shots to two groups of men. The first group was allowed to sleep only four hours a night for four nights, while the second group was allowed to sleep normally. Ten days after getting the flu shot, the sleep-deprived group had a significantly lower immune response than the normal-sleeping group. In fact, the under-sleepers actually produced less than half as many flu-fighting antibodies!

The bottom line: Pay attention to your sleep. Saying "I'll sleep when I'm dead" used to be a badge of honor among Type-A personalities, but the irony is that those who say that may well die sooner rather than later. They are not paying attention to the huge metabolic, hormonal, and anti-aging benefits of deep, restful sleep.

Sleep Recommendations: The Art and Science of Catching Forty Winks

We want you to make getting a good night's sleep—every night of the year—a priority. It's essential for your health, your longevity, your performance, and your waistline. And although people may vary in their individual sleep needs, we think seven hours a night is the magic number needed for optimal health. (Steven sleeps seven to eight hours, Jonny sleeps six.)

Some tips for better sleep that we've found helpful over the years include:

- *Keep the room dark.* Studies show that even dim light can disrupt melatonin production. Harvard sleep researcher Stephen Lockley notes that light at night is part of the reason so many people don't get enough sleep.
- *Keep the room cold.* Sleep experts say that the ideal temperature for sleep is around 68 degrees. A mild drop in body temperature helps induce sleep, and it's easier for that to happen if you're in a cooler room.
- *Never fall asleep with the TV on.* There's nothing soothing and restful about a subliminal soundtrack of news, infomercials, and reruns of the Kardashians. That TV soundtrack gets into your brain, disturbs your sleep, and frequently causes dreams of Thighmasters and Insanity. You may feel that you need the TV on to soothe you to sleep, but really, you don't. Try silence. You'll sleep better.

Not only is the *amount* of light important, but different *types* of lighting help you to wake up and to go to sleep:

- Wake up to bright light; it matches your cortisol surge in the morning and helps wake you. If you can get out in the sunlight first thing in the morning, that's awesome. If not, consider wide-spectrum bright lighting for the first thirty to sixty minutes after you wake in the morning.

- Use red-orange light before you go to sleep, especially if you suffer from insomnia. One to two hours before bedtime, wear red-orange glasses or turn your bedroom into a red-light room. Red light simulates sunset and bedtime for humans and stimulates your brain to produce melatonin and put you to sleep.
- Avoid white-background TV or computer screens one to two hours before going to bed as white light tells your primitive brain to wake up.

Smart Relationships

One of the most popular books of recent years—*The Blue Zones: Lessons for Living Longer from the People Who've Lived the Longest*—was written by a reporter, Dan Buettner, who traveled to four areas of the world called "Blue Zones": the Japanese island of Okinawa; Sardinia, Italy; the Nicoya Peninsula of Costa Rica; and Loma Linda, California, specifically, the Seventh-day Adventist community based there. (A fifth Blue Zone—the Greek island of Ikaria—was identified more recently.)

Blue Zones have the greatest concentrations of healthy centenarians in the world. These aren't folks just hanging on to life in hospitals or assisted living. They're largely robust, active people, typically living active lifestyles gardening, herding, or otherwise tending the land. Buettner wanted to see whether there were any commonalities among the people of the Blue Zones in an attempt to understand what the heck kept them so healthy into their ninth decades and beyond. After all, wouldn't it be great to learn their secrets?

The people of the Blue Zones did indeed have some things in common, but not as many as you might think. They didn't all eat the same diet (though none of them ate processed foods and they all ate a high-fiber diet). They certainly didn't belong to gyms, and they didn't take supplements. And while most were active, they didn't all do the same kinds of things. Ultimately, it turns out, there are very few elements related to diet or exercise or sleep or stress that are universal among all healthy, long-lived people.

Except one.

There happens to be one single category of human activity that is just about universal among every culture everywhere in the world in which people have generally great health and live a long time. It's as close a thing as we have to a "universal truth" about health. And it has almost nothing to do with what we eat, how we sleep, or how we exercise. If you put that universal truth on a wall-mounted plaque, it would read:

THERE IS NO HEALTH WITHOUT A STRONG SOCIAL FABRIC.

There's simply not a single long-lived society anywhere in the world that doesn't have a set of strong social connections. These can (and do) include family, community, places of worship, rituals, activities, and all the rest of the structures that accompany cohesive group living. Without that social structure, we might as well be sitting alone on a desert island where we will quietly burn out in a matter of years.

Psychologists have long used the term *emotional intelligence* as shorthand for the ability to handle interpersonal relationships empathetically; emotional intelligence is widely believed to be one of the keys to professional and personal success. Here, we use "emotional intelligence" to mean the sum total of everything in our lives that relates to our relationships with others, our relationship with our own emotions, and our ability to communicate. If we can harness the power of our emotions, we can use them to facilitate problem solving, communication, and—perhaps most important for our health—our connections to other people.

Our thoughts and emotions have powerful effects on our physiology. You may not be able to "think yourself thin," but you can certainly "think yourself sick." In fact, there's an entire legitimate field of science, known as *psychoneuroimmunology,* that studies how our thoughts influence our health, our immune systems, and our resistance to disease. What we think about—what we focus on and put our energy into—affects our blood pressure, our heart rate, the amount of hormones we release in our body, even our cholesterol levels!

A big part of what we're calling emotional intelligence is how we relate to and interact with others. It's hardly an accident that people in successful marriages live longer than singles. The University of North Carolina Alumni Heart Study found that having a partner during middle age is protective against premature death. Other research has shown that married people have a lower risk of developing cardiovascular disease.

The key, of course, to the "marriage advantage"—or, more correctly, the *relationship* advantage—is the quality and character of that relationship. All sorts of health benefits accrue to people in strong, generally healthy relationships, but a stressful marriage confers no benefits at all. "When we divide good marriages from bad ones," says author and historian Stephanie Coontz, "we learn that it is the relationship, not the institution, that is key." (For the record, Steven has been happily married for twenty-eight years and Jonny is in a long-term committed relationship.) In fact, for people who don't have many relationships, or whose relationships are weak, the risk of dying prematurely is between two and four times greater than for those who have strong social bonds; this is true regardless of race, age, physical health, smoking, alcohol use, physical activity, socioeconomic status, and even obesity.

We think a good case can be made that the health benefits of any successful relationship have a lot to do with the attention paid to something or someone outside ourselves. And there's some ingenious research that supports this theory. Back in the 1970s a Harvard psychologist named Ellen Langer gave all of the residents of a nursing home a plant. Half the residents were told that the plant would be taken care of by the nursing home staff, and the other half were told that the plant was their responsibility. The people who took care of the plant themselves had fewer doctor visits, better medical outcomes, better blood tests, and higher scores on virtually every measure of well-being that the researchers were able to come up with. Simply taking care of a plant improved their health significantly in measurable ways. And that's just a plant! Imagine what might happen when you take care of other people, volunteer, get involved in a charity or a shelter, or do anything else that takes the attention off yourself and contributes to the welfare of others.

"Human beings are not meant to live solitary lives," says John Rowe, the former chair of the MacArthur Foundation Research Network on Aging. "Talking, touch, and relating to others are essential to our well-being."

So what's the takeaway? We think it's clear: Every single study of healthy people shows that the No. 1 thing about them is that they're connected to others. They have friends—and we're not talking about Facebook "likes"; we're talking about real-life, face-to-face people whom they interact with and care about. Healthy people have relationships, and they care about things and put energy into things that make a difference to other people. Scientists would love to study healthy one-hundred-year-olds who live in isolation, but there's just one problem: They don't exist.

Some people defy every other "rule" of healthy living: They don't eat well. They smoke. They don't exercise. They take lousy care of their bodies. Yet by some miracle of the genetic lottery, they seem to live long and prosper.

But it's almost impossible to do that in isolation, to live long and well without connections to family or a spouse, or to social groups, or to a community, or to a religious institution, or to some other social entity that gives life meaning and purpose.

We've spent most of our adult lives studying people, and the more we learn, the more profound respect we have for how little we know.

We've both changed what we believe about food and exercise many times in our combined fifty-five years of experience in the health field. But there's one belief that we have both held, independently and consistently, for all of our professional lives: People want to contribute.

They want to make a difference. They want to have meaningful lives. They want it to matter that they were here. They want to do good.

Whether we're conscious of it nor not, whether we express it or not, whether we're successful at it or not, the truth is that the desire to contribute and make a difference to other people is at the core of what it means to be human. It's what makes life both fulfilling and beautiful. It's what the people of Okinawa call *ikigai*—a reason for being, a purpose.

If we had one overall health strategy to leave you with—a strategy that makes everything else you've learned in this book worthwhile—it would be this: *Find your purpose.*

And live in accordance with it, every single day. We hope this book has given you the tools to do just that.

Enjoy the journey.

Jonny and Steven

CHAPTER 10

Smart Recipes

HERE YOU'LL FIND MORE THAN fifty recipes that form much of our Smart Fat Solution Thirty-Day Plan. Steven, a trained chef and fellow-certified nutritionist, developed and fine-tuned all these recipes exclusively for this book (you can find additional recipes on our website at www.SmartFat.com). We hope these recipes will also inspire you to come up with your own variations; feel free to experiment and change flavors and ingredients, or prepare them with a cooking technique that works for you. (Just note that the preparation time, serving information, and, most importantly, nutritional content for each dish corresponds to the recipe as printed here.)

Before you get cooking, however, we'd like for you to do a little housecleaning—specifically, in your fridge and kitchen cabinets (and don't forget that junk drawer where you stash the leftover pieces of Halloween candy!). You know what to throw out—from dumb fats to sugary carbs and processed foods, we've armed you with loads of info on what not to eat and what not to put in your shopping cart.

You also need to know what you *should* have on hand to help you set up a truly smart kitchen. You'll find tips and suggestions on various ingredients within the recipes themselves, but let's focus on some that will allow you to put together a smart fat meal or snack with ease.

The Smart Pantry: Herbs and Spices

Flavor is as vital a part of the Smart Fat Solution as smart fat, fiber, and protein—because great flavors mean you'll stick with the smart fat way of eating. Great flavor also means great nutrition—and great health benefits. As we pointed out in Chapter 2, many herbs and spices have anti-inflammatory, anti-aging properties, which is why we use them liberally in our cooking.

Here's our "smart spice rack" list of dried herbs and spices, followed by a list of fresh flavors to have on hand, including a short-list of go-to herbs that are easy to grow at home, even if your thumb isn't green.

- Italian dried herb seasoning[†]
- Fines herbes
- Thyme
- Oregano
- Dill weed
- Ground paprika
- Ground cayenne pepper
- Crushed red pepper flakes
- Whole black peppercorns (for freshly ground black pepper)
- Curry spice blend
- Cinnamon
- Cardamom
- Sea salt

Fresh flavors to have on hand:

- Garlic
- Gingerroot

[†] Look for a combination of Italian herbs such as oregano, thyme, basil, rosemary, and marjoram. Avoid "seasoning" mixes, which may contain non-herb ingredients.

- Parsley
- Cilantro
- Basil
- Mint
- Rosemary

The last five in the list—parsley, cilantro, basil, mint, and rosemary—are easy to grow in containers or in a small garden patch (but watch out for invasive mint—it's almost *too* easy to grow! Its fresh flavor and versatility, however, can't be beat). One great thing about growing fresh herbs is that you can harvest what you don't use at season's end, dry or freeze it, or purée it with a little bit of extra-virgin olive oil and keep it on hand as a great pop of summer flavor, even in the middle of winter.

The Smart Pantry: Oils (and Smoke Points)

We're very careful about choosing the right oil for the right (cooking) task, because when heat is applied to oil, it can change—and *damage*—the makeup of otherwise beneficial substances. Use too much heat and you'll turn a smart fat into a dumb fat.

Take extra-virgin olive oil, for example—everybody's poster child for the best oil ever. Extra-virgin olive oil is made by simply crushing olives and extracting the juice. It's made without a hint of chemicals and industrial refinement and under temperatures that won't degrade the oil (that is, less than 86°F). People pay a lot more money for extra-virgin olive oil and then proceed to use it for *all* their cooking needs—including cooking at high heat.

Big mistake.

Think about it. Why did you pay such a high premium for extra virgin in the first place? It was to get all those spectacularly healthy olive polyphenols, undamaged by heat or chemicals. So why would you take this carefully made oil, just dripping with delicate and beneficial compounds, and then heat it to a high temperature that essentially destroys its makeup?

It doesn't make much sense, does it?

There's a term for the temperature at which oils begin to be damaged: the *smoke point*. When an oil is heated until it smokes, the valuable nutrients are damaged. Worse, the oil becomes harmful to ingest. If you take a smart fat—such as extra-virgin olive oil or unrefined coconut oil—and you cook it past its appropriate temperature tolerance, you've just taken a smart fat and made it into a dumb one.

So, pay attention to the temperature guide below, and never use an oil at a temperature that causes it to smoke. (Don't go nuts over this, though; if you happen to accidentally burn an oil from time to time, just take the pan off the heat, wipe it with a paper towel, and start over.)

What Oils to Have in Your Pantry

For cooking at high heat: We suggest you choose one or two oils for high-heat cooking—like avocado, pecan, extra-light olive oil, or ghee (clarified butter; see our recipe below for Beef Stew for instructions on how to make ghee). Of these, avocado and pecan oils are packed with nutrients and are smart fats; extra-light olive oil and ghee would be neutral fats.

For cooking at medium to high heat: Medium- to high-heat oils are the ones you'll probably use most of the time. (Steven recommends mainly medium- to high-heat oils for browning meat or poultry or for cooking vegetables.) Good choices for medium- to high-heat oils are virgin olive oil (not *extra* virgin), almond oil, hazelnut oil, and macadamia nut oil—all of which are smart fats!

For cooking at medium heat: Use nutrient-rich smart fat choices like extra-virgin olive oil and unrefined coconut oil.

For cooking at medium to low heat: Use virgin olive oil, unrefined sesame oil, and unrefined walnut oil.

For cooking at low heat: Use pistachio oil.

For salad dressings and drizzling for additional flavor (that is, no heat): Choose nutrient-rich oils, with extra-virgin olive oil leading the way. High-lignin flaxseed oil can also be used for drizzling or dressings (but never for cooking, *ever*). Other oils that work well for this

APPROPRIATE OILS FOR HIGH, MEDIUM, AND LOW HEAT	
COOKING HEAT	APPROPRIATE OIL
High heat (450–650°F)	Avocado oil, grapeseed oil, pecan oil, ghee (clarified butter), extra-light olive oil
Medium-high heat (375–449°F)	Virgin olive oil, almond oil, hazelnut oil, refined walnut oil, macadamia nut oil, refined coconut oil
Medium heat (325–374°F)	Extra-virgin olive oil, lard, butter, unrefined coconut oil
Medium-low heat (250–324°F)	Unrefined sesame seed oil, unrefined walnut oil
Low heat (225–249°F)	Pistachio oil

OILS, SMOKE POINTS, AND MAXIMUM COOKING TEMPERATURES		
OIL	SMOKE POINT	MAXIMUM COOKING TEMPERATURE
Almond oil	430°F	Medium high
Avocado oil	520°F	High
Avocado oil, virgin	400°F	Medium
Butter	350°F	Medium
Butter, clarified	485°F	High
Coconut oil, refined	400°F	Medium
Coconut oil, unrefined	350°F	Medium low
Grapeseed oil	485°F	High
Hazelnut oil	430°F	Medium high
Lard	380°F	Medium
Macadamia nut oil	400°F	Medium
Olive oil, virgin	420°F	Medium high
Olive oil, extra virgin	400°F	Medium
Olive oil, extra light	470°F	High
Pecan oil	470°F	High
Pistachio oil	250°F	Low
Sesame oil, unrefined	350°F	Medium low
Walnut oil, refined	400°F	Medium
Walnut oil, unrefined	320°F	Medium low

purpose include sesame, pistachio, and walnut oils. Extra-virgin olive, pistachio, and walnut oils are all smart fats.

See the charts for cooking heats and appropriate oils, and smoke points and maximum cooking temperatures. The bottom line: Use the right oil, but use it at the right temperature! That's just plain smart cooking!

Additional Smart Pantry Items

Broths: Organic and low-sodium vegetable, chicken, and beef broths.

Canned or jarred staples:† Beans (white, red, any variety you like) and lentils; artichoke hearts (packed in water or olive oil); wild salmon and sardines (packed in water or olive oil); whole, chopped, and crushed tomatoes; roasted red peppers; marinara sauce (organic, no added sugar); canned coconut milk.

Dark chocolate: Organic, at least 70 percent cocoa.

Grains: Wild rice, quinoa, steel-cut oats.

Coconut milk: Coconut milk products vary greatly. Canned coconut milk is thick and high in fat. Coconut milk beverage in a carton is much thinner and lower in fat. We use canned coconut milk for curries and sauces and carton coconut milk beverage for drinks, like protein shakes.

Nuts and nut butters: Almonds (whole and slivered), walnuts, pecans, pistachios, hazelnuts, and macadamia nuts. Tip: Buy nuts in bulk and freeze or store them in glass jars or stainless-steel containers. Almond butter, natural peanut butter.

Protein powder: Grass-fed and organic whey, organic soy or pea-rice; see our Smart Fat Shake recipe for more information.

Vinegars and sauces: Red wine vinegar, balsamic vinegar, hot chili sauce (such as Tabasco), gluten-free tamari.

Dairy items: Organic plain yogurt, Greek-style and regular; organic and unsweetened almond, soy, or coconut milk (for your Smart Fat Shake) or organic cow's milk; organic butter; Parmesan (or Parmigiano-Reggiano cheese); organic-fed, cage-free eggs.

Produce: The following items will keep well: organic lemons, limes, and oranges; onions; purple and sweet potatoes; carrots; celery. Tip:

---

† Look for BPA-free cans, or buy items in glass jars, if you can. Bisphenol A (BPA) is a potentially toxic compound that is found in the plastic lining of metal cans and in plastic bottles and storage containers. Though some manufacturers have stopped using it, it's still on store shelves. That's why we prefer pantry items that are in glass jars, as well as glass or stainless-steel storage containers.

Keep carrots and celery fresh and ready-to-eat by prepping and putting them into glass storage containers with a little bit of water to keep them fresh and crunchy.

Avocados are a smart fat staple! Buy three or four at a time and let them ripen on your kitchen counter. Once ripe (there should be a little give—but not too much—when you squeeze them), you have one to two days to use them. You can slow the ripening process by putting them in the fridge, but we recommend you eat them as soon as they're ready. Tip: Hasten the ripening process by putting an avocado in a paper bag with half an apple. It really works!

Poultry, meat, fish: Choose *clean protein:* organic, grass-fed, and wild-caught. Buy in bulk and freeze it. If you can't find it locally, see the resources at www.SmartFat.com.

A note on food safety and poultry, meats, and fish: Until recently, rinsing chicken, meat, and fish before cooking was a common instruc-

---

PRODUCE: ORGANIC OR NOT ORGANIC?

Are you wondering whether you should buy organic-everything when it comes to produce? You don't have to. Some items—such as onions, cabbage, asparagus, avocado, peas, and broccoli (a staple for us)—are generally free of heavy pesticides, but other items—especially those with thin, penetrable skins that we eat—are more vulnerable and you should spring for the organic versions.

Here are some produce items that you should buy organic: apples, strawberries, cherries, peaches, pears, celery, cherry tomatoes, potatoes, bell peppers, and greens such as spinach and lettuce. Check out the Environmental Working Group's complete and most updated lists of produce most likely to contain higher and lower levels of pesticide residue (the Dirty Dozen and the Clean Fifteen; www.ewg.org). The good news is that organic produce is increasingly available at competitive prices.

tion, but researchers have found that some home cooks inadvertently spread illness-causing bacteria in their kitchens and food-serving areas if they splash juices or contaminated water and do not sanitize sinks, counters, cutting boards, and other areas carefully after rinsing and patting dry these items. If you cook food to the proper temperature, you *should* kill off all bacteria; the problem is that we don't always cook food to a high enough temperature.

Exercise common sense when you handle raw poultry, fish and meat, and if you choose to rinse, be sure to clean the prep area carefully to avoid cross-contamination. (Unfortunately, it's a myth that organic, grass-fed animal products have less bacteria than conventionally raised products, but there is a silver lining: These animals are not given antibiotics, so any bacteria in their meat is much less likely to be drug-resistant. If you're treated for illness, the drugs you get will work!)

A note on cooking techniques: Proper rinsing and cooking to the proper temperature is one way to lower the risk of bacteria, but marinating poultry, meat, and fish before grilling also makes them safer. Marinating in an acidic solution (such as citrus juice, Italian dressing with vinegar, or teriyaki sauce with vinegar) naturally reduces the risk of producing heterocyclic amines—nasty, cancer-causing compounds that form when animal fats and juices hit the flames of a grill. That sizzling sound is nice, but the compounds that may form as a result are dangerous. Marinating reduces them by 80 percent! What's more, marinating with these acidic solutions means the meat will retain moisture better, preventing grilled food from drying out.

And Don't Forget to Stock the Freezer

Frozen fruits and veggies: Organic berries, cherries, and peaches (it's cheaper to buy frozen than fresh); organic vegetables; frozen spinach and kale leaves for your Smart Fat Shake.

Poultry, meat, fish: Buy it fresh and freeze it, or buy it frozen. You'll never run out of clean protein if you keep your freezer stocked!

Vacuum-packed frozen fish prevents most freezer burn and tastes much better than frozen fish in a loose bag.

Must-Have Kitchen Essentials

Finally, here's Steven's Top 20 list of must-have kitchen tools, pots, and pans. He makes good use of all of these when he prepares the recipes you're about to enjoy. Happy cooking—and happy eating!

1. Chef's knife (longer is better) and a smaller paring knife; kitchen scissors
2. At least two cutting boards
3. Sauté pans (medium and large; if you have only one, larger is better); avoid aluminum and cast iron—look for stainless steel or anodized aluminum, such as Calphalon; avoid pans with teflon and other plastic linings
4. Saucepans (small and medium)
5. Big soup pot (at least 8 quarts)
6. Strainer
7. Colander
8. Steamer
9. Measuring spoons
10. Glass measuring cups (1- and 2-cup)
11. Blender (Steven prefers Vita Mix)
12. Wooden spoons (square and oval)
13. Spatulas (one wide, one long and narrow)
14. Peeler, cheese grater, and micro planer for citrus zest
15. Food processor and egg beater
16. Oven-proof baking dish (9 by 13 inches)
17. Pie plate
18. Baking sheets, including rimmed baking sheet
19. Glass storage containers with tight-fitting plastic lids (don't store or cook your food in plastic)
20. Glass or metal mixing bowls

THE RECIPES

Breakfast

Smart Fat Shake

This is our basic protein-packed morning shake, with added smart fat and fiber. It's ideal when you don't have time to fix a full breakfast and also is a great quick lunch, snack, or dessert. See the box for tips on getting the most of your shakes, and check out our flavorful variations that follow. Also for variety, change the fruit or berry or the flavor of your protein powders— vanilla, chocolate, and strawberry.

You can smart-fat any protein shake you make by simply adding a tablespoon of nut butter, MCT oil, 1–2 tablespoons of chia seeds or flaxseed, or a tablespoon of nut oil, including coconut oil. For variety, you can change the fruit or berry, or the flavor of your protein powders between vanilla, chocolate, and strawberry.

Prep Time: 2 minutes
Serves: 1 (makes 2½ cups)

20 grams protein powder (1–2 scoops) (grass-fed and organic whey or organic soy or pea-rice)
8–12 ounces almond milk, unsweetened
1 cup frozen berries of your choice
1 handful frozen spinach or kale leaves
1 serving smart fat of your choice: 1 tablespoon almond butter, MCT oil; 1–2 tablespoons chia seeds or flaxseeds; or 1 tablespoon nut oil

Combine ingredients in a blender and process first at slow speed, then increase to the fastest setting.

SHAKE SMARTS

Whether you're making our basic Smart Fat Shake or one of our variations, here are a few tips:

- Remember: You can smart-fat any shake or smoothie by adding a tablespoon of nut oil, MCT oil, almond butter, or nut flour (ground nuts) or 1–2 tablespoons of chia seeds or flaxseed. Most smart fats will not change the fruity taste of your shake. Experiment with what you like best.

- If your protein powder contains less than 5 grams of fiber, add a fiber supplement like chia seeds or ground flaxseeds, Medibulk Thorne fiber, PaleoFiber, or Sunfiber to get at least that amount (5 extra grams of fiber).

- Use frozen, organic berries, cherries, or other fruit; you can purchase frozen organic items more cheaply than fresh, they're ready to use whenever you want them, and their frozen quality adds a refreshing texture to your shake.

- Freeze spinach and kale for shakes. Place fresh leaves in zippered plastic bags and keep them in the freezer along with your stash of frozen berries and you'll always have key ingredients on hand. (If kale leaves are particularly large, roughly chop them before freezing.) Note: You can also use fresh spinach and kale for your shakes, but we like frozen for convenience and texture.

- Once you make a shake, drink it right away. After 10–15 minutes the shake components start to separate and it loses the proper texture.

Smart Fat Shake:
Vanilla, Blueberry, and Spinach

Steven makes this shake most mornings. Substitute kale for spinach and use more liquid if you like your shake thinner. A cup of blueberries adds fiber (3.5 grams). Add an additional fiber supplement unless you're using a protein powder that has at least 5 grams of fiber. You can smart-fat this or any variation of our Smart Fat Shake.

2 scoops Vanilla Smart Fat Protein Powder†
8-12 ounces unsweetened almond milk
1 cup frozen organic blueberries
1 handful frozen spinach leaves
1 tablespoon almond butter

Combine ingredients in a blender and blend until smooth, about 1 minute.

Nutrient Content Per Serving

Calories: 325	Protein: 21.5 grams
Fiber: 13 grams	Carbs: 26.7 grams
Sodium: 226 milligrams	Fat: 14.1 grams

Vanilla, Cherry, and Kale Shake

Here is another favorite, to alternate with the blueberries.

2 scoops Vanilla Smart Fat Protein Powder†
10 ounces unsweetened almond milk
1 cup frozen cherries (organic)
1 handful frozen chopped kale
1 tablespoon chia seeds

Combine ingredients in a blender and blend until smooth, about 1 minute.

Nutrient Content Per Serving

Calories: 325	Protein: 22.5 grams
Fiber: 14.7 grams	Carbs: 34 grams
Sodium: 290 milligrams	Fat: 10.8 grams

---

† Or use any organic whey protein powder. Our Smart Fat® Protein Powder includes 6 grams of fiber. If yours does not, remember to add an additional fiber supplement.

Smart Fat Shake: Chocolate and Strawberry

We love the chocolate and strawberry combo–delicious!

2 scoops Chocolate Smart Fat Protein Powder[†]

8-12 ounces unsweetened almond milk

1 cup frozen organic strawberries

1 tablespoon MCT oil

Combine ingredients in a blender and blend until smooth, about 1 minute.

Nutrient Content Per Serving

Calories: 348	Protein: 22 grams
Fiber: 10.3 grams	Carbs: 16 grams
Sodium: 270 milligrams	Fat: 19.5 grams

Smart Fat Shake: Chocolate, Cherry, and Spinach

Chocolate and cherries are great together, and you'll never know the spinach is there.

2 scoops Chocolate Smart Fat Protein Powder[†]

10 ounces unsweetened almond milk

1 cup frozen organic cherries

1 handful frozen spinach leaves

1 tablespoon almond butter

Combine ingredients in a blender and blend until smooth, about 1 minute.

Nutrient Content Per Serving

Calories: 376	Protein: 27.5 grams
Fiber: 12.5 grams	Carbs: 31.5 grams
Sodium: 292 milligrams	Fat: 14 grams

[†] Or use any organic whey protein powder. Our Smart Fat Protein Powder includes 6 grams of fiber. If yours does not, remember to add an additional fiber supplement.

Omelet with Sweet Onion, Red Bell Pepper, and Kale

This is a wonderful way to put eggs back on the menu. It's quick and easy—and it fills the kitchen with an irresistible herb fragrance. Have it for breakfast, lunch, or dinner. Always use cage-free, organic eggs for clean protein. If you have a local source, take advantage of the nutrition and terrific taste of farm-fresh eggs.

Prep Time: 10 minutes

Serves: 2

6 large organic-fed, cage-free eggs

4 teaspoons virgin olive oil, divided

½ medium sweet onion, diced

¼ teaspoon sea salt

⅛ teaspoon ground black pepper

½ teaspoon dried Italian herbs

1 medium red bell pepper, thinly sliced

2 cups fresh kale (or spinach)

2 tablespoons grated Parmesan cheese

2 tablespoons fresh chopped Italian parsley (for garnish)

Heat a sauté pan to medium-high, add 2 teaspoons oil, and sauté onion with salt, pepper, and herbs for 2 minutes. Reduce heat to medium, add bell pepper and spinach, and sauté for 2 minutes. Meanwhile, whisk eggs in a bowl.

When sautéed veggies are nearly cooked, combine them with eggs in bowl. Quickly wipe sauté pan with a paper towel, add remaining 2 teaspoons olive oil, then add egg and vegetable mixture into the hot pan. Lift edges of the egg and tilt the pan to allow uncooked egg to pour toward the edge of the pan and cook. When nearly done, sprinkle grated cheese over the eggs, fold omelet in half, sprinkle with parsley, and serve.

Nutrient Content Per Serving

Calories: 372	Protein: 23 grams
Fiber: 3 grams	Carbs: 16.3 grams
Sodium: 567 milligrams	Fat: 25 grams

Frittata

A tasty frittata works for any meal, just like an omelet. (Eggs aren't just for breakfast!) This one is simple to make and attractive to serve.

Prep Time: 10–15 minutes
Baking Time: 15–20 minutes
Serves: 2

1 tablespoon virgin olive oil
2 cups sliced mushrooms (button or shiitake)
¼ teaspoon sea salt
¼ teaspoon ground black pepper
1 teaspoon dried Italian herbs
1 cup quartered artichoke hearts, drained
4 medium green onions, diced
2 cups fresh spinach
1 small tomato, diced
6 large organic-fed, cage-free eggs
½ cup organic whole milk (or organic sour cream)
½ cup grated Gruyère cheese (divided in half)

Preheat oven to 350°F.

Bring an oven-proof 9–10-inch sauté pan to medium heat. Add oil, then mushrooms, salt, black pepper, and Italian herbs. Cook, stirring occasionally, 3–5 minutes, until mushrooms are soft. Add artichoke hearts, green onion, spinach, and tomato; heat and stir occasionally until spinach wilts, another 2 minutes.

Whisk eggs in a bowl, stir in milk and half the cheese. Then stir in mushroom mixture. Pour contents back into the sauté pan, top with remaining cheese, and heat for 1 minute on the stovetop so the eggs begin to cook.

Transfer to the oven. Bake 15–20 minutes. The frittata should have the texture of custard–trembling and barely set; if you cook until the top is firm, it is overcooked. After baking, turn the oven to broil 2–3 minutes, just enough to lightly brown the top of the frittata. Serve immediately–if left in the pan, it will overcook.

Nutrient Content Per Serving

Calories: 644	Protein: 34 grams
Fiber: 7 grams	Carbs: 25 grams
Sodium: 644 milligrams	Fat: 42.5 grams

Smart Fat Steel-Cut Oatmeal

This simple-to-prepare hot cereal is low in sugar and provides the fiber and protein needed to sustain you through the day.

Stovetop Prep Time: 3 minutes, plus 20–30 minutes simmering time
Microwave Prep Time: 3 minutes, plus 8 minutes cooking time
Serves: 1

1 cup water
¼ cup steel-cut oats
⅛ teaspoon ground cinnamon
Pinch of sea salt
1 scoop Vanilla Protein Powder (with 10–12 grams protein)
½ cup almond milk (or organic cow's milk)
2 tablespoons slivered almonds (or any chopped nuts)
½ cup fresh berries (or other sliced fruit)

If preparing in a saucepan, bring water to a boil. Add oats, cinnamon, and salt; reduce heat to low and simmer 20–30 minutes, or until oats are tender but still chewy. Five minutes before serving, stir in protein powder and milk. Add nuts and fruit.

If preparing in a microwave, combine water, oats, cinnamon, salt, and protein powder in a large glass bowl. Microwave 8 minutes. Serve with almond milk, nuts, and fruit.

Nutrient Content Per Serving

Calories: 332	Protein: 20 grams
Fiber: 7.6 grams	Carbs: 37.5 grams
Sodium: 263 milligrams	Fat: 12 grams

Snacks and Appetizers

Cucumber with Smoked Oysters and Avocado

Instead of having oysters with crackers, try them with thinly sliced cucumber. Crunchy and refreshing! Oysters are smart to eat as they are loaded with zinc, protein, arginine, and omega-3 fats. If you can't find canned smoked oysters in olive oil in your store, you may need to order them online. Don't buy oysters canned in cottonseed oil (a dumb fat!).

Prep Time: 5 minutes
Serves: 2

3 ounces smoked oysters (canned in olive oil), drained
1 medium ripe avocado
1 tablespoon lemon juice
⅛ teaspoon sea salt
¼ teaspoon ground paprika
1 medium garlic clove, minced or pressed
2 tablespoons finely chopped fresh cilantro (or Italian parsley)
1 medium cucumber, thinly sliced
Dashes of hot sauce (optional)

Drain oysters. Mash avocado and mix with lemon juice, salt, paprika, garlic, and cilantro. Spread cucumber slices on a serving plate. Add a spoonful of avocado mixture to each slice, then top with one to two smoked oysters. For a touch of heat, add a dash of your favorite hot sauce.

Nutrient Content Per Serving

Calories: 261	Protein: 10.3 grams
Fiber: 6.7 grams	Carbs: 18.6 grams
Sodium: 315 milligrams	Fat: 18.8 grams

Asian Pear, Gorgonzola Cheese, Walnuts, and Raspberries

Instead of cheese and crackers, try this mouth-watering, healthier alternative. You can substitute any variety of pear or apple for the Asian pear and use your favorite type of cheese and any kind of berry. Tip: Slice the cheese so that you have enough for each slice of fruit. For a nicer presentation, use walnut halves.

Prep Time: 5 minutes
Serves: 2

1 medium Asian pear, sliced into bite-size pieces
2 ounces gorgonzola cheese, thinly sliced (see tip above)
1-2 ounces walnuts, halves preferred
¼ cup fresh berries of your choice

Spread Asian pear slices on a serving platter and top each with a piece of cheese, walnuts, and berries.

Nutrient Content Per Serving

Calories: 309	Protein: 10.2 grams
Fiber: 7.4 grams	Carbs: 20 grams
Sodium: 513 milligrams	Fat: 23 grams

Crab Avocado Dip

This delicious dip tastes best fresh, so make what you'll eat on the spot. Serve with sliced cucumber or bell peppers or baby endive leaves. As with the crab recipe below, using good-quality crab meat–the freshest tasting you can find–is essential! Freshly caught and cracked crab is obviously the best, but refrigerated crab sold in many stores can be excellent. Be sure to check the expiration date if using refrigerated crab.

½ pound lumped crab meat, drained
2 tablespoons lemon juice
1 avocado, mashed
¼ teaspoon sea salt
⅛ teaspoon black pepper

⅛ teaspoon cayenne pepper (to taste)

1 tablespoon finely chopped Italian parsley

Combine all ingredients and serve immediately.

Nutrient Content Per Serving

Calories: 115	Protein: 10 grams
Fiber: 3 grams	Carbs: 4.4 grams
Sodium: 445 milligrams	Fat: 6.7 grams

Lump Crab and Mango-Avocado Salsa

This elegant, flavorful salsa makes a super appetizer or light meal.

Prep Time: 20–30 minutes

Serves: 4

Crab Mixture

½ pound lump crab meat, drained

½ medium red bell pepper, finely diced

2 medium green onions, finely diced

½ medium lemon, juiced

Mango-Avocado Salsa

1 medium mango, peeled and diced

1 medium ripe (but firm) avocado, diced

½ medium lemon, juiced

⅛ teaspoon sea salt

⅛ teaspoon ground cayenne pepper

¼ cup chopped cilantro

1 large seedless cucumber, sliced into ⅛-inch slices

Combine crab meat with bell pepper, green onion, and lemon juice. In a separate bowl, combine mango, avocado, lemon juice, salt, cayenne pepper, and cilantro. Spread cucumber slices over a serving platter and top each with 1 tablespoon crab mixture, then 1 tablespoon mango-avocado salsa. Serve immediately.

Nutrient Content Per Serving

Calories: 167	Protein: 11 grams
Fiber: 4.8 grams	Carbs: 18 grams
Sodium: 375 milligrams	Fat: 7 grams

Guacamole with Jicama and Red Bell Pepper

Guacamole is a staple for Steven and his wife, Nicole. They buy three to four avocados every week, and half go to making some variation of this dish. Avocados are one of their favorite smart fats!

Prep Time: 10 minutes
Serves: 4

1 medium jicama root, peeled and sliced (see below)
1 medium red bell pepper, sliced into 1-inch thin strips
Juice of 1 lime
1 large avocado
¼ sweet onion, minced
½ cup chopped fresh cilantro
⅛ teaspoon sea salt
⅛ teaspoon ground black pepper
Ground cayenne pepper to taste (⅛ to ¼ teaspoon)
Cilantro and hot sauce for garnish

Prepare the jicama: Peel away the brown skin to expose the white flesh, then slice into thin chip-sized pieces. Toss jicama and bell pepper pieces with a quarter of the lime juice. Place on a serving plate.

Cut avocado into small pieces and mix in a serving bowl with remaining lime juice, onion, cilantro, salt, black pepper, and cayenne pepper. Garnish with cilantro sprigs. Add hot sauce to taste.

Nutrient Content Per Serving

Calories: 148	Protein: 2.5 grams
Fiber: 11.7 grams	Carbs: 21.6 grams
Sodium: 84.8 milligrams	Fat: 7 grams

Salads

Avocado, Cucumber, and Garbanzo Salad

Garbanzo beans, or chickpeas, are packed with taste and nutrition, and we make good use of them in the Smart Fat Solution. You can use ones that are canned if you don't cook your own—just rinse them well. This salad is easy to put together; enjoy it as either a side dish or a light meal. Lightly toasting the almonds (or any raw nuts you use in recipes) always brings out their flavor.

Prep Time: 10 minutes
Serves: 2

1 cup cooked garbanzo beans, rinsed and drained
½ medium seedless cucumber, chopped
2 medium tomatoes, chopped
½ cup Italian parsley, chopped
2 garlic cloves, minced
⅛ teaspoon sea salt
⅛ teaspoon ground black pepper
2 tablespoons extra-virgin olive oil
1 tablespoon red wine vinegar
1 medium avocado, sliced
1-2 tablespoons slivered almonds, lightly toasted

Combine garbanzo beans, cucumber, tomatoes, and parsley (reserve 2 tablespoons parsley for garnish) in a salad bowl. Whisk together garlic, salt, pepper, oil, and vinegar in a small bowl and add to salad. Toss well and divide between two plates. Garnish each salad with avocado, almond slivers, and remaining parsley. Serve immediately.

Nutrient Content Per Serving

Calories: 462	Protein: 11.5 grams
Fiber: 13.4 grams	Carbs: 40 grams
Sodium: 195 milligrams	Fat: 31.2 grams

Home-cooked beans freeze well in small portions in their cooking liquid. Make a big batch, divide into 1- or 2-cup portions, and freeze. Defrost in the refrigerator or microwave as needed.

Shrimp, Fennel, and Cannellini Bean Salad with Orange Vinaigrette

Canned beans are convenient in a recipe like this one, though home-cooked beans will taste even better.

Prep Time: 15-20 minutes
Serves: 2

Shrimp Marinade

1 medium orange, juiced (see instructions)

1 teaspoon ground paprika

1 teaspoon sea salt

1 pound large shrimp, peeled and deveined

Salad

1 tablespoon almond oil

1 medium fennel bulb, cut into 1-inch slices

⅛ teaspoon sea salt

2 cups arugula

4 cups organic, mixed salad greens

1 cup cooked cannellini beans, rinsed and drained

Dressing

2 tablespoons extra-virgin olive oil

1 tablespoon red wine vinegar

2 medium garlic cloves, minced

1 tablespoon orange rind, grated

1 tablespoon orange juice

⅛ teaspoon ground black pepper

Garnish

1 tablespoon grated Parmesan cheese

6 cherry tomatoes, sliced in half

Before juicing the orange, grate 1 tablespoon rind and set aside; after juicing, reserve 1 tablespoon orange juice. Both will be used for the dressing.

Combine remaining orange juice, paprika, and sea salt in a large bowl and add shrimp; marinate for at least 10 minutes or up to several hours in the refrigerator.

Heat a sauté pan over medium heat. Add almond oil, then sauté sliced fennel with salt, stirring occasionally for 3 minutes. While fennel is cooking, drain shrimp and add to sauté pan, cover, and stir occasionally until shrimp are pink and cooked, 3-4 minutes. (Discard marinade.)

Place salad ingredients in a large serving bowl. Whisk together all dressing ingredients in a small bowl. Toss salad with dressing. Add shrimp and fennel to salad and garnish with grated cheese and cherry tomatoes.

Nutrient Content Per Serving

Calories: 604	Protein: 57 grams
Fiber: 10.6 grams	Carbs: 35.2 grams
Sodium: 721 milligrams	Fat: 27.1 grams

White Bean Salad

Beans make an excellent cold salad when mixed with herbs and crunchy veggies. Refrigerate beans before you use them as you'll want them cold for this side dish, which also can be a light lunch. Use any white bean of your choice. Just make sure they're firm (not mushy) so that they hold up in this salad.

Prep Time: 10-15 minutes
Serves: 2

2 cups cooked white beans, drained and refrigerated

2 tablespoons virgin olive oil

½ medium onion, diced

¼ teaspoon sea salt

¼ teaspoon ground black pepper

1 teaspoon dried Italian herbs

2 medium celery stalks, diced

4 medium garlic cloves, minced

1 medium carrot, grated

½ cup Italian parsley, finely chopped

2 tablespoons grated Parmesan cheese

Place beans in a large salad bowl. Heat a sauté pan over medium heat, then add oil, quickly followed by onion, salt, pepper, and herbs. Cook 2 minutes, stirring occasionally; add celery and cook another 2 minutes. Stir in garlic and cook 1 minute more. Remove pan from heat and add to beans in the salad bowl. Mix in grated carrot, parsley, and Parmesan cheese. Serve immediately, or refrigerate and serve later.

Nutrient Content Per Serving

Calories: 380	Protein: 57 grams
Fiber: 12 grams	Carbs: 35.2 grams
Sodium: 506 milligrams	Fat: 27.1 grams

Smart Vinaigrette Dressing

Steven uses a variation of this versatile dressing all the time. It's great with salads, but you can also use it to smart-fat your favorite raw or steamed veggies. This recipe makes four 2-tablespoon servings.

2 tablespoons balsamic vinegar (or red wine vinegar with lighter nut oils)

1 tablespoon white wine

5 tablespoons extra-virgin olive oil (vary by using avocado oil or your favorite nut oil)

½ teaspoon dried thyme

¼ teaspoon sea salt

¼ teaspoon fresh ground black pepper

2 medium garlic cloves, finely minced

½ to 1 teaspoon Dijon mustard (optional)

Combine ingredients and serve.

Nutrient Content Per Serving

Calories: 125	Protein: 0.1 gram
Fiber: 0.1 gram	Carbs: 1.3 grams
Sodium: 120 milligrams	Fat: 14 grams

Soups

Borscht

This classic Slavic winter soup is delicious, hearty, and colorful. Nearly all borscht served in Russia includes beef and makes a meal, but typically in Western countries we make a vegetarian version and serve it before the main dish. You can prepare our recipe with or without beef (grass-fed). If you're making a vegetarian version, just skip the first step (browning the beef) and proceed with the rest of the recipe. Note: If you can't find organic sour cream, use nonfat, because if you can't eat clean, eat lean!

Prep Time: 20 minutes
Simmering Time: 30 minutes
Serves: 6

4 medium beets
2 tablespoons virgin olive oil
1½ pounds grass-fed beef chuck, cut into bite-size pieces (optional)
1 medium white onion, diced
¼ teaspoon sea salt
½ teaspoon ground black pepper
½ teaspoon dried dill
1 teaspoon caraway seeds
2 medium carrots, ¾-inch cubed
2 medium celery stalks, chopped
2 cups purple potatoes (or baby red-skinned potatoes), cut into bite-size pieces
2 cups coarsely chopped red cabbage
4 medium garlic cloves, diced
2 cups chopped tomatoes (or 1 can [15-ounce] chopped tomatoes)
6 cups low-sodium organic vegetable or beef broth

Garnish
½ cup organic sour cream (or conventional nonfat sour cream) or organic plain yogurt
¼ cup diced chives

Bring 6 cups of water to a boil. Rinse beets and trim off the roots and tops. Drop beets into boiling water for 1 minute (to help remove the skins). Allow to cool, then peel. Cut two beets into ¾-inch cubes; grate the other two beets. Set aside.

Heat a large saucepan to medium-high heat, add olive oil and beef, stirring occasionally until all pieces are browned, about 5 minutes. Remove beef and set aside.

Add onion to the pan and sauté with salt, pepper, dill, and caraway seeds for 2-3 minutes, until seeds are slightly yellow to golden. Add cubed and grated beets to the pan and stir. Then add carrots, celery, potatoes, cabbage, garlic, tomatoes, meat, and broth. Bring to a gentle boil, then reduce heat and simmer 30 minutes. (If you're making this with beef, skim off any foam that forms on the surface.)

Serve in individual bowls and garnish with a dollop of sour cream or yogurt and chives.

Nutrient Content Per Serving

Calories: 530	Protein: 40 grams
Fiber: 5 grams	Carbs: 24.6 grams
Sodium: 694 milligrams	Fat: 30 grams

Here's a great habit to get into: If you have a little extra time on the weekends, make up a big batch of soup that you can enjoy during the week. Also, soups and stews develop more flavor for a day or two after cooking, so they're ideal as leftovers.

Soup of the Week

Here's a typical soup that Steven prepares on weekends for lunch during the week. Note: Use organic marinara sauce in a jar, or visit our website for our recipe (www.SmartFat.com).

Prep Time: 20 minutes
Simmering Time: 10 minutes
Serves: 6-8

2 tablespoons virgin olive oil
1 medium sweet onion, diced

½ teaspoon sea salt

½ teaspoon ground black pepper

1 teaspoon dried Italian herbs

1 cup sliced mushrooms

2 medium carrots, diced

2 medium celery stalks, diced

1 medium sweet potato, peeled and cut into ¾-inch cubes

1 cup marinara sauce

4 cups low-sodium organic vegetable or chicken broth

2 cups chopped broccoli (bite-size pieces)

15-ounce can white or red beans, rinsed and drained

15-ounce can garbanzo beans, rinsed and drained

Heat a large stockpot to medium-high heat and add oil, onion, salt, black pepper, and herbs. Cook 2-3 minutes, stirring occasionally, until onion is translucent. Then stir in mushrooms, carrots, celery, and sweet potatoes. Reduce heat to medium and cook another 5 minutes, stirring a few times. Add marinara sauce and broth and bring to a gentle boil. Reduce heat to low, add broccoli and beans, and simmer 10 minutes.

Nutrient Content Per Serving

Calories: 243	Protein: 11.6 grams
Fiber: 10 grams	Carbs: 38 grams
Sodium: 653 milligrams	Fat: 5.7 grams

Butternut Squash Soup with Ginger and Fennel

This fragrant, delicate soup is especially good for fall and early winter when butternut squash—a great source of fiber and beta-carotene—is in season. The savory flavors of gingerroot and fennel go perfectly with squash.

Baking Time: 35-45 minutes

Prep Time: 20 minutes

Simmering Time: 10 minutes

Serves: 6

1 medium butternut squash (2–3 pounds)

2 tablespoons almond oil (or your favorite nut oil)

½ medium onion, chopped

½ teaspoon sea salt

½ teaspoon ground black pepper

1 tablespoon peeled and grated gingerroot

1 teaspoon curry powder

1 cup coarsely chopped fennel (bulb only–save the feathery leaves for garnish)

¼ cup white wine

2 cups low-sodium organic vegetable or chicken broth

1 cup organic half-and-half or cream (or organic whole milk)

Preheat oven to 400°F. Cut squash in half lengthwise, scoop out seeds, and bake facedown on a lightly oiled baking dish for 35–45 minutes, until soft enough to scoop out the flesh with a spoon. Set flesh aside.

Heat a large saucepan over medium-high heat and add oil. Sauté onion with salt and pepper until onion is translucent, 2–3 minutes. Add gingerroot, curry powder, and fennel. Heat 2–3 minutes, stirring occasionally. Add wine; after 30 seconds add stock and all but ¼ cup of the cream. Stir and remove from heat. Purée in a blender or food processer.

Add squash pulp to puréed ingredients. Blend or process until smooth, 1–2 minutes. Return to saucepan and heat through for about 10 minutes.

To serve, pour into individual bowls, garnish with fennel leaves, and add a swirl of cream.

Nutrient Content Per Serving

Calories: 167	Protein: 3.3 grams
Fiber: 5.8 grams	Carbs: 19.4 grams
Sodium: 401 milligrams	Fat: 8.7 grams

MAIN DISHES

Poultry

Roasted Chicken with Mediterranean Herbs

You can change up the flavor profile of your roast chicken by varying the herb rub you use. Italian seasonings are terrific, but for a French twist use herbes de Provence (featuring savory, thyme, rosemary, marjoram, oregano, and optionally lavender). A roast chicken is one of the simplest dishes to prepare—just leave enough time for baking.

Prep Time: 10 minutes
Baking Time: 65-75 minutes
Serves: 4

3- to 4-pound whole organic, cage-free chicken
3 tablespoons virgin olive oil
1 tablespoon dried Italian herbs
1 teaspoon sea salt
½ teaspoon ground black pepper

Preheat oven to 425°F. Rinse chicken and pat dry with paper towels. Rub skin all over with oil, herbs, salt, and pepper.

Place chicken in a roasting pan on middle rack of the oven for 5 minutes, then reduce heat to 400°F for 60-70 minutes (until meat thermometer inserted deep into the thigh reads 160°F). Switch oven to broil for an additional 3-5 minutes or until skin is golden. (Final temperature should be 165°F.) Remove from oven and let sit 10 minutes for juices to redistribute before carving. Transfer carved pieces to a serving platter and serve.

Nutrient Content Per Serving

Calories: 546	Protein: 48 grams
Fiber: 0 grams	Carbs: 0 grams
Sodium: 605 milligrams	Fat: 40 grams

Moroccan Chicken Stew

Loaded with flavor and packed with spices, this exotic-tasting dish is surprisingly simple to make. To vary the recipe, try other proteins, such as lamb or steak, and don't hesitate to try other vegetables, too.

Prep and Cooking Time: 25-30 minutes
Simmering Time: 10 minutes
Serves: 4

1 ½ pounds boneless chicken thighs, cut into ½-inch pieces
3 tablespoons virgin olive oil
1 medium white onion, chopped
¼ teaspoon sea salt
3 medium celery stalks, chopped
1 medium carrot, chopped
3 medium zucchini, chopped
1 tablespoon curry powder (or 2 teaspoons dried turmeric and
  1 teaspoon ground cumin)
1 teaspoon dried paprika
½ teaspoon ground cinnamon
⅛-½ teaspoon ground cayenne pepper (to taste)
15-ounce can chopped tomatoes (or 2 cups fresh)
2 cups chopped cabbage
1 cup low-sodium chicken or vegetable stock
1 cup canned coconut milk (or organic whole milk)
¼ cup chopped fresh mint leaves
1 tablespoon lemon juice
1 ounce (about one handful) chopped or slivered almonds, toasted

Heat a large pot over medium-high heat, add oil, and sauté chicken 5-7 minutes, stirring occasionally, until lightly browned. Remove chicken and set aside. In the same pan, add onion and salt, reduce heat to medium, and sauté with a few stirs for 2 minutes. Add celery, carrot, zucchini, and spices and cook for another 2 minutes, stirring occasionally.

Stir in tomatoes, cabbage, browned chicken, and stock. Once bubbling, reduce heat to low, add coconut milk and simmer 10 minutes. While simmering, toast almonds in a separate pan over medium-low heat for 1–2 minutes, until heated but not browned. Set aside.

Stir in mint and lemon juice and serve in bowls. Garnish with toasted almonds.

Nutrient Content Per Serving:

Calories: 650	Protein: 39 grams
Fiber: 4.1 grams	Carbs: 49 grams
Sodium: 672 milligrams	Fat: 22 grams

Turkey Meatballs

These taste great served with ratatouille or marinara sauce (see our recipes for both at www.SmartFat.com).

Prep Time: 10–15 minutes
Cooking Time: 10–15 minutes
Serves: 3

½ medium onion, minced

3 green onions, diced

2 eggs, beaten

4 tablespoons marinara sauce

½ cup grated Parmesan cheese

½ teaspoon sea salt

½ teaspoon black pepper

1 teaspoon dried Italian herbs

¼ cup garbanzo bean flour (or ¼ cup mashed garbanzo beans)

¼ cup Italian parsley, chopped

1 pound ground cage-free, organic-fed turkey (preferably from breast meat)

3 tablespoons virgin olive oil (for sauté)

Combine ingredients in a bowl and form into 1- to 1¼-inch balls. Heat a large sauté pan to medium heat. Add oil, then sauté turkey meatballs until lightly browned, turning every 2 minutes or so. Once browned (this will take about 10–12 minutes), reduce heat to low, cover and heat for another

2-4 minutes or until the meatballs are cooked through. If you don't have a large pan, do this in two batches. Do not overcrowd the pan.

Nutrient Content Per Serving

Calories: 483	Protein: 39 grams
Fiber: 2.4 grams	Carbs: 12 grams
Sodium: 839 milligrams	Fat: 33.5 grams

You may wonder why our poultry recipes don't necessarily specify skinless chicken or turkey. After all, most "diets" frown upon eating crispy skin. With the Smart Fat Solution, if you are using organic-fed, cage-free poultry—that is, clean protein—you may eat the skin; if not, skip it. Once again, if you can't eat clean, eat lean.

Sautéed Turkey Loins with Italian Herbs

This delicious dish is very easy to make. You can substitute chicken thighs for turkey loins.

Prep and Cooking Time: 15 minutes
Serves: 3

1 pound turkey loins, cut into 1-inch strips

1 tablespoon virgin olive oil

1 teaspoon dried Italian herbs

½ teaspoon sea salt

¼ teaspoon ground black pepper

1 teaspoon paprika

⅛ to ¼ teaspoon ground cayenne (optional)

1 tablespoon chopped parsley

In a bowl, combine turkey strips with oil, spices, and herbs; mix well. Heat a sauté pan to medium-high. Sauté turkey, turning occasionally, until lightly browned on all sides, 5-8 minutes. Serve with steamed broccoli seasoned with Smart Fat Vinaigrette or Smart Fat Butter Sauce.

Nutrient Content Per Serving

Calories: 203	Protein: 37 grams
Fiber: 0 grams	Carbs: 0 grams
Sodium: 472 milligrams	Fat: 5.4 grams

Chicken with Pecan-Herb Crust

Chicken with a nut crust is especially tasty. This recipe calls for pecan oil, but you can use almost any nut for the crust. Just match the oil with the nut you use.

Prep Time: 20–25 minutes
Baking Time: 20–25 minutes
Serves: 4

4 boneless organic-fed, cage-free chicken breasts
    (about 4 ounces each)
1 large organic-fed, cage-free egg
1 cup coarsely ground pecans
½ teaspoon sea salt
1 teaspoon dried thyme (or Italian herbs or fines herbes)
⅛ teaspoon black pepper
4 medium garlic cloves, minced
1 teaspoon pecan oil

Preheat oven to 425°F. Lightly coat a baking dish with nut oil. (Tip: Dip a paper towel in oil and rub the dish to coat.)

Rinse chicken breasts, then pat dry with paper towels. Beat the egg in a bowl, set aside. Heat a sauté pan to medium; lightly toast the ground pecans with salt, thyme, pepper, and garlic for 1–2 minutes. Transfer ¼ of nut mixture to a plate. Dip one chicken breast at a time in the egg, then press into the nut mixture so that both sides are coated. Place breasts in oiled baking dish. (Discard any leftover egg and nut mixture.)

Bake 20–25 minutes, until tender and flaky.

Nutrient Content Per Serving

Calories: 390	Protein: 39 grams
Fiber: 2.5 grams	Carbs: 4.7 grams
Sodium: 395 milligrams	Fat: 24 grams

Tandoori Chicken

This tastes wonderful and cooks quickly, but plan in advance because it needs at least 4 hours to marinate. Tip: Prepare the marinade in the morning or the evening before, and marinate the chicken all day; then pop in the oven when you get home.

Prep Time: 20 minutes
Marinade Time: 4–24 hours
Serves: 4

2 pounds organic-fed, cage-free chicken thighs (or any chicken parts)
1 medium lemon (organic)
½ medium onion, diced
1 cup plain organic, full-fat yogurt
2 teaspoons ground paprika
1 teaspoon ground cayenne pepper
1 tablespoon freshly grated gingerroot (or 1 teaspoon ground ginger powder)
1 teaspoon ground curry spice (or ground turmeric)
½ teaspoon sea salt
½ teaspoon ground black pepper
1 teaspoon ground paprika
1 medium lemon peel, finely diced
2 tablespoons chopped cilantro (or Italian parsley)

Lightly score chicken surface with a small, sharp knife (this will allow the marinade to penetrate the chicken) and put in a large bowl. Cut lemon in half and squeeze juice from both halves over chicken, while straining out the seeds (do not discard lemon halves). Allow chicken to marinate in lemon juice 5-10 minutes.

In a smaller bowl, combine yogurt, onion, paprika, cayenne, ginger, turmeric, salt, and pepper. Pour marinade over chicken, cover, and marinate 4-24 hours. Dice squeezed lemon halves and set aside.

When marinating is done, set oven to broil. Remove chicken from marinade and place in a lightly oiled oven-proof dish (discarding extra marinade). Sprinkle paprika and diced lemon peel over chicken and broil on the top rack, approximately 4-6 inches from the heat, for 5-8 minutes, turning once until each side is lightly browned. Reduce heat to 400°F and bake another 10–15 minutes or until meat thermometer inserted in the thickest portion reaches 165°F. Sprinkle with chopped cilantro and serve.

Nutrient Content Per Serving

Calories: 535	Protein: 42 grams
Fiber: 0.5 gram	Carbs: 7 grams
Sodium: 505 milligrams	Fat: 36.6 grams

Middle Eastern Chicken Sauté

The cardamom and ginger flavors are terrific in this dish. You can use steak, fish, or tofu if you want a different protein. (Fish and tofu cook more quickly than chicken or steak.)

Prep and Cooking Time: 15–20 minutes
Serves: 2

2 tablespoons virgin olive oil
1 medium onion, chopped
½ teaspoon sea salt
¼ teaspoon ground black pepper
1 pound organic-fed, cage-free chicken thighs
½ teaspoon ground cardamom
1 tablespoon freshly grated gingerroot
  (or 1 teaspoon powdered ginger)
⅛ teaspoon cinnamon
2 medium garlic cloves, diced

Heat a sauté pan to medium-high heat, add oil, then onion, salt, and black pepper, stirring occasionally for 2 minutes. Add chicken and heat, stirring occasionally until lightly browned, 4–5 minutes. Reduce heat to medium-low and add cardamom, ginger, cinnamon, and garlic; simmer 3–5 minutes until chicken is fully cooked (thickest piece is cooked through or 165°F with a meat thermometer).

Nutrient Content Per Serving

Calories: 626	Protein: 40 grams
Fiber: 1 gram	Carbs: 6.5 grams
Sodium: 765 milligrams	Fat: 48.5 grams

Chicken Satay Skewers with Cabbage Wraps

You can prepare this meal in advance, making it a perfect dish to share with guests. You control the heat on this traditionally spicy dish. Make it hot–use your favorite chili sauce–or not and make it mild. You can grill the chicken or prepare it indoors under the broiler. Metal skewers work best; if using wood skewers, soak them in water for 30 minutes in advance to avoid charring.

Prep Time: 40-45 minutes
Cooking Time: 15-20 minutes
Serves: 4

Chicken Satay

2 pounds chicken thighs, cut into bite-size pieces
2 tablespoons coconut oil (divided in half)
2 tablespoons peeled and grated gingerroot (divided in half)
4 medium garlic cloves, minced (divided in half)
⅛ teaspoon ground cayenne pepper
½ lime, juiced
1 tablespoon tamari

Vegetable Mixture

Remaining coconut oil, gingerroot, and garlic cloves
1 medium onion, thinly sliced
¼ teaspoon sea salt
⅛ teaspoon ground black pepper
½ teaspoon ground paprika
1 cup snow peas
1 medium red bell pepper, thinly sliced

Almond Butter-Coconut Milk Sauce

4 tablespoons almond butter (or natural peanut butter)
½ cup canned coconut milk
½-2 tablespoons hot chili sauce (Tabasco, Cajun, or hot Thai chili
sauce–adjust to heat preference)

Cabbage Wraps

8 large green cabbage leaves (from a large head of cabbage)

Marinate chicken: Place chicken pieces in bowl. Add 1 tablespoon each coconut oil and ginger and half the garlic to chicken. Add cayenne pepper, lime juice, and tamari sauce. Marinate 30-40 minutes, stirring occasionally.

Prepare vegetable mixture: Heat sauté pan to medium heat; add remaining coconut oil with onion, salt, pepper, and paprika. Sauté 3-4 minutes until onions are translucent. Add remaining ginger and garlic with snow peas and bell pepper, and heat another 3-4 minutes until veggies are still crisp but tender. Remove from heat.

Make sauce: Combine almond butter, coconut milk, and hot chili sauce in a small saucepan. Heat and stir over medium heat. Add 2-3 tablespoons as needed of milk to get the proper thickness for a sauce. Once sauce is hot, remove from heat.

Prepare cabbage wraps: Place 2 inches of water at the bottom of a steamer pot and bring to a boil. Discard the outer layer of cabbage leaves (contact with the environment makes them tough and dirty). Peel away the next eight large cabbage leaves, taking care to minimize tearing. Add separated cabbage leaves loosely to steamer pot and steam until tender, 8-10 minutes.

If grilling, preheat grill. Thread chicken on metal skewers. Grill 10-12 minutes, turning every 3-4 minutes, until lightly browned. If broiling, set oven to broil. Thread chicken on metal skewers and broil 6-8 inches under the heat 10-15 minutes, turning every 4-5 minutes, until lightly browned.

During the last 5 minutes of grilling/broiling, reheat the vegetables and sauce if needed.

To serve and assemble: Arrange serving dishes with cabbage leaves, almond butter-coconut sauce, veggie mix, and chicken satay (remove from skewers). Each diner places a cabbage leaf on a plate, adds a scoop of veggies, then chicken satay, then drizzles with sauce. Roll cabbage leaf like a burrito. You can eat with a knife and fork or with your fingers. (Offer extra napkins!)

Nutrient Content Per Serving

Calories: 536	Protein: 52 grams
Fiber: 5 grams	Carbs: 16 grams
Sodium: 633 milligrams	Fat: 30 grams

Meat Dishes

Roasted Grass-Fed Bison and Root Vegetables

Bison is easy to roast and it's increasingly available from many butchers and markets. If you can't find bison, use grass-fed beef. This dish makes a great meal, but the baking time varies, so rely on the meat thermometer to know when it is done.

Prep Time: 10–15 minutes
Baking Time: About 45 minutes
Serves: 4

2 pounds bison sirloin or tenderloin (or grass-fed beef);
    avoid chuck as it is too tough
1 tablespoon dried Italian herbs
½ teaspoon sea salt
½ teaspoon ground black pepper
4 medium garlic cloves, minced
2 tablespoons virgin olive oil (divided in half)
1 large sweet onion, chopped into 1-inch chunks
4 medium beets, peeled and cut into ¾-inch cubes
4 medium carrots, cut into ¾-inch cubes
1 tablespoon fines herbes
½ teaspoon sea salt
¼ teaspoon ground black pepper
2-3 tablespoons chopped fresh herbs of your choice
    (such as Italian parsley or basil)

Preheat oven to 400°F. With a sharp knife, carefully slice away most of the tough silver skin (the thin, membrane layer covering parts of the roast).

In a bowl, mix Italian herbs, salt, pepper, garlic, and 1 tablespoon olive oil. Rub over the roast. Mix the chopped onion, beets, and carrots in a separate bowl with the fines herbes, additional salt and pepper, and remaining 1 tablespoon oil.

In a roasting pan, add bison and circle with cubed vegetables. Roast in oven 20 minutes, then reduce heat to 375°F. Roast about 15 minutes more, until bison temperature is 140-145°F when measured with a meat thermometer. *It is helpful to use a meat thermometer to avoid overcooking (and an overly tough roast).*

Remove bison from pan, place on a cutting board, and cover with foil. The bison will continue to cook while resting. Return pan with vegetables to the oven and raise temperature to 400°F. Bake vegetables until tender, another 10-15 minutes. Just before removing vegetables from the oven, slice bison roast and confirm that it is medium-rare (pink). If too rare for your taste, roast another 5-10 minutes in the oven, but don't overcook.

Place roast slices on a serving platter, encircle with cooked vegetables, and garnish with fresh herbs.

Nutrient Content Per Serving

Calories: 528	Protein: 66 grams
Fiber: 4.6 grams	Carbs: 18.5 grams
Sodium: 817 milligrams	Fat: 20 grams

Sirloin Steak Chili

Make sure to always choose grass-fed meat for this terrific chili. Try sirloin, but it tastes just as good if you use ground turkey. Either way, all chili tastes even better left over, once the flavors have melded.

Prep Time: 20-25 minutes

Simmer Time: 5-10 minutes

Serves: 4

2 tablespoons virgin olive oil

1 medium onion, chopped

½ teaspoon sea salt

¼ teaspoon ground black pepper

1 teaspoon dried oregano

1 teaspoon ground paprika

2 pounds grass-fed, organic sirloin steak, cut into ½-inch cubes

2 medium carrots, diced

1 medium celery stalk, diced

2 medium poblano chilies, stem and seeds removed, diced

¼-½ teaspoon crushed red pepper (to taste)

4 medium garlic cloves, diced

1 cup water

2 cups chopped tomatoes (or 1 can [15-ounce] chopped tomatoes)

**3 cups (or 2 [15-ounce] cans) cooked pinto beans, rinsed and
drained**

½ cup chopped fresh cilantro

Heat a large saucepan on medium-high heat, add oil, then onion, salt, black
pepper, oregano, and paprika. Sauté 1 minute. Add steak cubes, stirring
occasionally another 2–3 minutes, until lightly browned. Add carrots and
celery; sauté another 2 minutes, stirring a few times.

Add chilies, crushed pepper, garlic, water, and tomatoes. When chili is
bubbling, stir in pinto beans. When bubbling again, reduce heat and simmer
10 minutes. Just before serving, stir in chopped cilantro.

Nutrient Content Per Serving

Calories: 745	Protein: 82 grams
Fiber: 14 grams	Carbs: 46 grams
Sodium: 476 milligrams	Fat: 23 grams

Marinated Flank Steak over Mixed Green Salad

Serve this flavorful steak over a salad. As always, grass-fed beef is the only
way to go! Steven prefers using artichoke hearts in glass jars with olive oil,
but canned artichokes in water are easier to find.

Prep Time: 10 minutes
Marinating Time: 30–60 minutes
Grill Time: 10 minutes
Serves: 4

1½ pounds grass-fed and organic flank steak

2 tablespoons balsamic vinegar

2 tablespoons virgin olive oil

1 tablespoon tamari

4 medium garlic cloves, minced

¾ teaspoon sea salt

½ teaspoon ground black pepper

½ teaspoon dried Italian herbs

8 cups mixed organic greens

1 cup cherry (or grape) tomatoes, sliced in half

4 cups artichoke hearts, quartered and drained

2 tablespoons red wine vinegar

4 tablespoons extra-virgin olive oil

2 medium garlic cloves, minced

In a large bowl, combine vinegar, oil, tamari, and garlic with steak. Refrigerate 30–60 minutes, turning the steak occasionally.

Preheat grill or turn oven to broil. Remove meat from marinade, season with salt, pepper, and Italian herbs. Grill or broil 3–6 minutes per side until internal temperature is 140–150°F. Transfer steak to a cutting board and let rest covered 5–10 minutes for juices to distribute evenly throughout the meat.

Meanwhile, mix salad greens with cherry tomatoes and artichoke hearts and toss with vinegar, oil, and minced garlic dressing. Serve on individual plates. Slice steak into ¼- to ½-inch slices and serve over salad greens.

Nutrient Content Per Serving

Calories: 483	Protein: 44 grams
Fiber: 10.6 grams	Carbs: 25 grams
Sodium: 743 milligrams	Fat: 24 grams

Tamari sauce is a gluten-free Japanese sauce similar to soy sauce with a rich, distinctive taste that pairs wonderfully with other flavors, including garlic and Italian herbs. If you've never used it before, we think you're going to discover a wonderful condiment that you'll want to use again and again.

Grilled Lamb Chops

Grill these chops or cook them under the broiler. Either way, lamb is a delicious source of protein. You can find various cuts of lamb (bone-in generally takes a little longer to cook). Loin chops are tenderer than shoulder chops. As with beef, choose organic and grass-fed.

Prep and Cooking Time: 30 minutes

Serves: 2

1 tablespoon virgin olive oil

1 tablespoon red wine vinegar

1 tablespoon chopped fresh rosemary

1 tablespoon chopped fresh mint leaves
1 medium shallot, minced
¼ teaspoon sea salt
⅛ teaspoon ground black pepper
1 pound lamb chops

Combine oil, vinegar, rosemary, mint, shallot, salt, and black pepper in a bowl. Rub chops with oil and herb combination and let sit at least 10 and up to 60 minutes. Grill or broil 4–5 minutes per side until desired doneness.

Nutrient Content Per Serving

Calories: 550	Protein: 68 grams
Fiber: 0 grams	Carbs: 0 grams
Sodium: 488 milligrams	Fat: 29 grams

Steak Kebobs with Pineapple, Onion, and Bell Pepper

Use grass-fed beef, chicken, or shrimp for these scrumptious kebobs (sirloin or tenderloin works nicely for kebobs). Their savory flavors go wonderfully with the natural sweetness of pineapple, peppers, and onions.

Prep Time: 20 minutes
Marinating Time: 30 minutes
Grilling/Broiling Time: 10–15 minutes
Serves: 2

For the marinade:
4 medium garlic cloves, minced
1 teaspoon hot chili sauce
1 medium lime, juiced
½ teaspoon sea salt
¼ teaspoon ground black pepper
1 teaspoon ground paprika
1 tablespoon almond oil

1 pound grass-fed tenderloin steak, cut into 1-inch cubes
1 cup pineapple cubes (large enough to go on skewers)
2 medium bell peppers (1 red and 1 green), cut into 1-inch squares
½ medium sweet onion, cut into 1-inch pieces

2 cups shredded cabbage
1 tablespoon extra-virgin olive oil
1 tablespoon red wine vinegar

Combine marinade ingredients in a small bowl and set aside. In a larger bowl, combine steak cubes with pineapple, bell pepper, and onion. Cover with marinade, mix well, and marinate in the refrigerator at least 30 minutes (preferably 1-2 hours), stirring occasionally. For the kebobs, metal skewers work best; if using wood skewers, soak them in water, while steak is marinating, to avoid charring.

Preheat grill or turn on broiler. Thread skewers with cubes of steak, pineapple, bell pepper, and onion. Brush additional marinade over each skewer, then discard marinade (do not baste skewers with leftover marinade while cooking).

If grilling: Cook 10-12 minutes, turning skewers 2-3 times. If broiling: Place kebobs on roasting pan 4-6 inches from heat, for 12-15 minutes. Internal temperature of steak should be 140-150°F. (If cooking chicken, internal temperature should be 165°F.)

Toss shredded cabbage with oil and vinegar. Serve kebobs on top of cabbage.

Nutrient Content Per Serving

Calories: 566	Protein: 53 grams
Fiber: 5.7 grams	Carbs: 27 grams
Sodium: 455 milligrams	Fat: 28 grams

Beef Stew

This classic stew is packed with protein and fiber. It's the perfect dish to make on a leisurely weekend and enjoy all week. You can buy organic, clarified butter, sold as ghee (make sure you purchase plain ghee, without spices).

Prep Time: 15-20 minutes
Simmering Time: 2-3 hours
Serves: 6

2 pounds grass-fed beef chuck, cubed
2 tablespoons organic clarified butter (ghee)
1 teaspoon sea salt
½ teaspoon ground black pepper

1 medium yellow onion, chopped

2 tablespoons chopped fresh rosemary

2 tablespoons chopped fresh thyme

2 tablespoons chopped fresh sage

3 cups low-sodium organic beef broth

15-ounce can chopped tomatoes

3 medium carrots, cut into ½-inch pieces

3 medium celery stalks, cut into ½-inch pieces

2 medium zucchini squash, cut in chunks

1 medium yellow squash, cut in chunks

Heat a large soup pot to medium-high heat, add butter to melt, then sauté beef, turning to brown on all sides; season with salt and pepper as it cooks. Note: If needed, do this in two batches to ensure all meat browns evenly. Transfer browned beef to a plate and set aside.

Sauté onion until translucent, about 3 minutes. Add rosemary, thyme, and sage and cook 1 minute more. Add beef broth and tomatoes, bring to a gentle boil, then add meat and any juices that have accumulated on the plate; reduce heat to low. Simmer, covered, 2–3 hours, stirring occasionally, and skimming off any foam on the surface.

Forty-five minutes before serving, add carrots, celery, and squash and simmer until vegetables are tender.

Nutrient Content Per Serving

Calories: 470	Protein: 33 grams
Fiber: 3.6 grams	Carbs: 12.5 grams
Sodium: 894 milligrams	Fat: 32 grams

Clarified butter, or ghee, is easy to make yourself: Place organic butter in a heavy saucepan and melt slowly over medium heat. Bring to a boil, then reduce heat and allow it to simmer 5 minutes, or until mixture is light gold in color. (Cooking time depends on the quantity of butter you are using.) Remove the pan from the heat and let butter cool slightly. Skim the foam from the top and discard. Slowly pour remaining oil into a container and save, discarding the milky solids at the bottom of the pan. What makes clarified butter so great is its higher smoke point. It will keep in the refrigerator for several months.

Seafood

Depending on where you live, it can be a challenge to find fresh fish. If you catch it yourself, you know it's fresh! (Steven lives in Florida, where at local fish markets, he's lucky to find the catch of the day most days.) But when you buy it, choose carefully. The skin should be moist. Ask to smell the fish before it's wrapped. If it smells too fishy, don't buy it—it should smell fresh like the ocean.

Baked White Fish with Orange Marinade

Fish is delicious baked—which happens to be one of the easiest ways to prepare it!

Prep Time: 10 minutes
Marinade Time: 5-10 minutes
Baking Time: 20 minutes
Serves: 2

1 tablespoon organic butter
1 medium orange for juicing
1 pound firm white fish (sole, cod, snapper, or tilapia)
½ teaspoon sea salt
¼ teaspoon ground black pepper
¼ teaspoon paprika
¼ cup Italian parsley, chopped

Preheat oven to 400°F. Coat the bottom of an oven-proof baking dish with butter.

Before juicing orange, cut two slices (to be served with cooked fish) and set aside. Juice the orange and marinate fish 5-10 minutes in juice, turning a couple of times.

Remove fish from marinade and season each side with salt, black pepper, and paprika. Add to baking dish and sprinkle with chopped parsley. Bake about 20 minutes. The fish should be tender and flake easily. Serve with a slice of fresh orange.

Nutrient Content Per Serving
_____

Calories: 343   Protein: 56 grams
Fiber: 0 grams   Carbs: 0 grams
Sodium: 751 milligrams Fat: 12 grams

Crab Cakes with Quinoa

Wait until you try crab cakes with quinoa instead of bread crumbs–awesome!

Prep Time: 20 minutes
Baking Time: 20 minutes
Serves: 4

⅓ cup uncooked quinoa

⅔ cup water or low-sodium vegetable stock

2 tablespoons virgin olive oil

1 cup diced onion (about ½ medium onion)

¼ teaspoon sea salt

2 medium celery stalks, diced

1 medium carrot, grated

1 teaspoon dried thyme

1 teaspoon ground paprika

1 pound crab, drained (refrigerated)

2 large organic, cage-free eggs, beaten

½ lemon rind, grated (use organic lemon)

½ lemon, juiced

2 tablespoons salted butter, divided into 8 portions

Rinse quinoa in a strainer, drain, then combine with water or stock in a saucepan and bring to a boil. Reduce heat to low, cover and cook 10 minutes. Turn off heat and keep covered. After about 10 minutes, quinoa should be tender (al dente) with a little white sprout popping from half the grains. Drain and set aside.

Preheat oven to 375°F. Butter an oven-proof dish and set aside.

Heat a sauté pan to medium-high heat, add virgin olive oil, then onion and salt; sauté 2–3 minutes, stirring occasionally, until onion is translucent. Reduce heat to medium, add celery, carrot, dried thyme, and paprika; cook 3–4 minutes until carrot and celery have softened to al dente (don't overcook).

In a large bowl, gently mix together quinoa, sautéed vegetables, crab, beaten eggs, lemon rind (grate the rind off half the lemon before juicing), and lemon juice. Divide and form into 8 cakes, about ¾- to 1-inch thick. Place crab cakes in baking dish, top each cake with ¼ tablespoon butter, and bake 20 minutes. If desired, broil for the final 3 minutes to lightly brown.

Nutrient Content Per Serving

Calories: 297	Protein: 26 grams
Fiber: 1.7 grams	Carbs: 12 grams
Sodium: 795 milligrams	Fat: 16 grams

When a recipe calls for grated or chopped citrus rind (lemon or orange, for instance), it's essential to use organic fruits to avoid pesticides that collect in the skin of sprayed fruit.

Coconut Milk Curry with Shrimp and Broccoli

Coconut curry is a popular dish in Steven's house, and not just because it features so many healthy ingredients. The Indian flavors are terrific, plus you can use any protein (shrimp, fish, chicken, tofu, or steak) and match with your favorite veggie combinations, such as cauliflower or peppers.

If preparing with chicken or steak, brown the pieces on all sides with onions 4–5 minutes early in the cooking process and continue cooking them while the rest of the ingredients are added to the pan.

Prep and Cooking Time: 25–30 minutes
Serves: 3

1½ cups hot water
¾ cup brown rice
1 tablespoon coconut oil
1 medium onion, chopped
¼ teaspoon sea salt
¼ teaspoon ground black pepper
1 tablespoon peeled and grated gingerroot

1 tablespoon curry powder

1 teaspoon ground paprika

⅛ to ½ teaspoon ground cayenne pepper
   (to taste, from mild to hot)

2 cups sliced broccoli

1 pound large or jumbo shrimp, peeled and deveined

2 medium garlic cloves, diced

12 ounces canned coconut milk

2 tablespoons chopped fresh cilantro or Italian parsley

Combine water and rice in pot, bring to a boil, then simmer 25-35 minutes until rice is cooked. (Rice brands vary, so follow package directions.)

Heat a large sauté pan to medium heat, add coconut oil, then onion, salt, and black pepper, and cook 3-4 minutes until onions are translucent. Add ginger, curry, paprika, and ground cayenne, stir, and heat another 2-3 minutes. Add broccoli, shrimp, and garlic, stirring occasionally until shrimp turn pink, 3-5 minutes. Reduce heat to low, stir in coconut milk, cover and simmer 5 minutes. Stir in fresh cilantro and serve over rice.

Nutrient Content Per Serving

Calories: 663	Protein: 39 grams
Fiber: 5.5 grams	Carbs: 56 grams
Sodium: 710 milligrams	Fat: 29 grams

Ceviche

For ceviche, very fresh fish–snapper, bass, sole, grouper, or flounder–is a must. Ceviche isn't cooked with heat, but it isn't raw fish, either. It is cured as it marinates by the natural acids found in lime or lemon juice. Steven prefers marinating 4 hours, but recipes say anything from 1 to 8 hours. It depends upon your palate and whether you like your fish lightly or fully cured ("cooked").

Prep Time: 20 minutes

Marinating Time: 1 to 8 hours

Serves: 4

**1 pound fresh snapper or other fresh fish, bone and skin removed,
cut into ½-inch cubes**

**½ cup freshly squeezed lime juice (enough to cover the fish when
marinating in a bowl)**

½ teaspoon sea salt

1 medium avocado, cut into ½-inch cubes

2 medium green onions, diced

½ medium yellow or red bell pepper, finely diced

¼ cup chopped fresh cilantro

¼ teaspoon sea salt

¼ teaspoon ground black pepper

⅛ teaspoon ground cayenne pepper

3-4 tablespoons freshly squeezed tangerine or lemon juice

1 tablespoon extra-virgin olive oil

**1 medium jicama, peeled and sliced into ¼-inch chips
(or sliced cucumber and bell pepper)**

Marinate snapper pieces in lime juice and salt until it is opaque when you cut through the thickest piece, about 4 hours. Twenty minutes before serving, combine avocado, green onion, bell pepper, tomato, cilantro, salt, black pepper, cayenne pepper, freshly squeezed tangerine juice, and olive oil in a serving bowl. Stir gently to mix well.

Drain snapper and add to avocado mixture. Use jicama and sliced veggies to dip.

Nutrient Content Per Serving

Calories: 291	Protein: 25.5 grams
Fiber: 11 grams	Carbs: 0.5 gram
Sodium: 379 milligrams	Fat: 12 grams

Broiled Oysters with Walnut, Parmesan Cheese, and Parsley Crust

If you can find fresh-off-the-boat oysters, this recipe takes full advantage of their remarkable flavor. Or, purchase refrigerated oysters. As with purchasing refrigerated crab, check the expiration date and go for the freshest ones you can find.

Prep Time: 10-15 minutes
Cooking Time: 10 minutes
Serves: 2

1 teaspoon almond oil or hazelnut oil
1 pint fresh, chilled oysters
½ cup walnuts
¼ cup Parmesan cheese
¼ cup Italian parsley
1 large egg, organic-fed, cage-free
Hot chili sauce (optional)

Set oven to broil with a rack positioned 4-6 inches from heat. Oil an oven-proof casserole dish (with almond or hazelnut oil–*avoid walnut oil as it may smoke with broiling*).

Drain oysters and pat dry with a paper towel. (If not completely fresh, marinate in citrus juice for 5 minutes, then drain and dry.)

Blend walnuts in a food processor or blender until they make a chunky meal. Then add cheese and parsley and blend just enough to mix together. Transfer the coating to a large plate.

Beat the egg in a bowl. Dip each oyster to coat with egg, then gently roll in the coating to evenly cover each side. Place in prepared casserole dish. Repeat with each oyster, and sprinkle the remaining coating over the top of the dish before broiling.

Broil about 10 minutes, until oysters and crust are lightly browned.

Nutrient Content Per Serving

Calories: 367	Protein: 21 grams
Fiber: 2 grams	Carbs: 16 grams
Sodium: 601 milligrams	Fat: 25 grams

Salmon with Smart Lemon-Butter Sauce

It's time for a *smart* butter sauce! This recipe was developed to serve with salmon, but you can use this sauce with many dishes, varying the fresh or dried herb to complement the dish. Use the best-quality organic butter you can find.

Prep Time: 10 minutes
Baking Time: 10 minutes
Serves: 4

Smart Lemon-Butter Sauce

1 tablespoon salted organic butter
1 tablespoon virgin olive oil
½ tablespoon grated organic lemon rind
½ tablespoon lemon juice
1 medium garlic clove, minced
¼ teaspoon dried dill weed (or other herb/spice of your choice)

Salmon with Smart Lemon-Butter Sauce

1½ to 2 pounds king, silver, or red salmon fillets
2 tablespoons freshly squeezed lemon or orange juice
½ teaspoon sea salt
¼ teaspoon ground black pepper

To make the lemon-butter sauce: Combine all ingredients in a pan and heat over medium heat until bubbling. Remove from heat.

To make the salmon: Preheat grill or broiler. Marinate salmon in citrus juice 5–10 minutes, turning occasionally, then drain. Sprinkle salmon with salt and pepper, then brush on 2 tablespoons of Smart Lemon-Butter Sauce. Broil 4–6 inches from heat or grill 8–12 minutes, just until fish flakes (about 10 minutes for a 1-inch-thick piece of salmon). Do not overcook.

Nutrient Content Per Serving

Calories: 382	Protein: 45 grams
Fiber: 0 grams	Carbs: 1.2 grams
Sodium: 419 milligrams	Fat: 21 grams

Baked Halibut with Almond Crust

Nut-crusted fish is delicious and loaded with smart fat. If you can't find fresh halibut, look for vacuum-packed, frozen halibut fillets. After they thaw, marinate in 1 cup orange juice and 1 teaspoon salt for 10 minutes.

Prep Time: 10 minutes
Baking Time: 20 minutes
Serves: 2

3 teaspoons organic butter, divided into thirds
Two 8-ounce halibut fillets
⅓ cup almonds
⅓ teaspoon sea salt
¼ teaspoon ground black pepper
1 organic-fed, cage-free egg

Preheat oven to 400°F. Lightly butter oven-proof dish with 1 teaspoon butter.

In a food processor, blend almonds, salt, and black pepper to the texture of coarse flour. Put half the mixture on a plate.

Beat egg in a shallow bowl. Dip halibut fillets in egg, then coat each side with almond mixture. Place in baking dish. Place 1 teaspoon butter on each fillet. Bake 20 minutes, until flaky.

Nutrient Content Per Serving

Calories: 448	Protein: 54 grams
Fiber: 2.5 grams	Carbs: 5 grams
Sodium: 512 milligrams	Fat: 23 grams

Vegetarian Dishes

Mushroom-Nut Pâté

This dish is incredibly rich, thanks to the nuts and mushrooms. It's great with shiitake mushrooms, but button mushrooms are very good too. Serve with a lightly steamed vegetable, a light salad, or both.

Prep Time: 25-30 minutes
Baking Time: 25-30 minutes
Serves: 4

- **1 tablespoon pecan oil**
- **1 medium sweet onion, diced**
- **4 cups diced shiitake or button mushrooms**
- **1 cup cooked chopped spinach (thaw frozen spinach or use 7 cups raw spinach)**
- **¼ teaspoon black ground pepper**
- **½ teaspoon sea salt**
- **1 teaspoon dried thyme**
- **½ cup port wine**
- **6 large organic-fed, free-range eggs**
- **1 cup finely chopped nuts (almonds, pecans, hazelnuts)**
- **½ cup grated Gruyère or Parmesan cheese**

Preheat oven to 400°F. Grease loaf pan with olive oil or line with parchment.

Heat pecan oil in a sauté pan over medium-high heat and add onion, cooking 1 minute. Add mushrooms, spinach, black pepper, salt, and Italian herbs; sauté 5 minutes, stirring occasionally and cooking until mushrooms have softened. Reduce heat to low, add port, and stir. Heat until the bottom of the pan is still moist but most of the port has evaporated. Set aside.

In a large bowl, mix eggs, nuts, and mushrooms, then pour mixture into prepared loaf pan. Bake 25-30 minutes until a toothpick inserted in center comes out clean. Remove from oven and let sit 5-10 minutes before serving. Slice and serve like meatloaf.

Nutrient Content Per Serving

Calories: 482	Protein: 26 grams
Fiber: 6 grams	Carbs: 19.5 grams
Sodium: 641 milligrams	Fat: 32.5 grams

Lentils are a fasting-cooking legume, are incredibly nutritious, and come in a variety of colors—for instance, yellow, red, brown, and black. Red lentils cook the quickest and are great with curries. Brown lentils hold their shape the best and work well for salads.

Lentil Curry

Serve these curried lentils alongside the next two recipes—Vegetable Korma and Raita—for a fabulous, Indian-inspired feast. If you can locate poppadum (chickpea wafers) at a specialty grocery store, they're an excellent accompaniment.

Prep and Cooking Time: 30 minutes
Serves: 4

1 cup red lentils

1 cup water

1 cup low-sodium organic vegetable broth

2 tablespoons coconut oil

1 medium sweet onion, diced

2 medium celery stalks, diced

1 tablespoon peeled and grated fresh gingerroot

1 tablespoon curry powder

½ teaspoon ground paprika

⅛ teaspoon ground cayenne pepper

2 medium garlic cloves, diced

¼ cup canned unsweetened coconut milk

Rinse and drain lentils. Combine lentils, water, and broth in a medium pot and bring to a boil. Reduce heat to low and simmer 20–25 minutes, until lentils are cooked but not soft. Set aside. (You may not need to drain them again if they absorb all the liquid.)

Meanwhile, heat oil in a sauté pan over medium heat. Add onion and cook 2–3 minutes until softened, stirring occasionally. Then add celery, ginger, curry powder, paprika, cayenne pepper, and cook 5 minutes more, stirring from time to time. Add garlic, reduce heat to low, then combine sauté mixture and coconut milk with lentils, stir and simmer another 5 minutes.

Nutrient Content Per Serving

Calories: 286	Protein: 14.5 grams
Fiber: 8.3 grams	Carbs: 34 grams
Sodium: 180 milligrams	Fat: 11 grams

Vegetable Korma

A korma is a curry thickened with yogurt or cream. Add the yogurt after removing the dish from the heat because heat will curdle the yogurt. Curries are packed with nutrients, anti-aging compounds–and flavor.

Prep and Cooking Time: 30 minutes

Serves: 4

2 tablespoons pecan oil (or any nut oil)

1 medium onion, diced

1 tablespoon peeled and minced fresh gingerroot

½ teaspoon sea salt

2 cups chopped cauliflower

2 cups diced okra (fresh or frozen)

8-ounce can tomato sauce (or 1 cup chopped tomatoes)

2 tablespoons curry powder

¼ teaspoon ground cayenne pepper (use more or less, to taste)

4 medium garlic cloves, minced

1 cup frozen green peas

1 red bell pepper, chopped

1 cup plain organic yogurt

¼ cup chopped fresh cilantro (for garnish)

¼ cup toasted pistachio nuts, chopped (for garnish)

Heat a skillet over medium-high heat. Add oil, then onion, ginger, and salt, stirring occasionally until onion is soft, about 3 minutes. Add cauliflower, okra, tomato sauce, curry powder, and cayenne pepper; reduce heat to medium and cook about 5 minutes. Add garlic, peas, and red bell pepper.

Reduce heat to low, cover, and simmer 10 minutes. Remove from heat, stir in yogurt, and serve, garnishing with cilantro and pistachio nuts.

Nutrient Content Per Serving

Calories: 256	Protein: 10 grams
Fiber: 7.8 grams	Carbs: 28 grams
Sodium: 657 milligrams	Fat: 13 grams

Raita

Raita is a wonderful, cool cucumber-yogurt dish served with curry or other spicy foods.

Prep Time: 5–10 minutes

Serves: 4

1 cup organic yogurt (low-fat or full-fat)

½ medium cucumber, diced

¼ cup finely diced red onion

2 tablespoons chopped fresh cilantro

¼ teaspoon sea salt

¼ teaspoon ground coriander

¼ teaspoon cumin seed (or ground cumin)

Combine all ingredients in a serving bowl. Garnish with a few sprigs of cilantro.

Nutrient Content Per Serving

Calories: 36	Protein: 3 grams
Fiber: 0.5 gram	Carbs: 6 grams
Sodium: 39 milligrams	Fat: 1 gram

Wild Mushroom Soufflé

Don't panic when you see the word "soufflé"—there's nothing complicated about this down-to-earth dish, which makes for a very satisfying vegetarian meal. Use any variety or combination of wild mushrooms, such as oyster or shiitake. Tip: When making a soufflé, bake in the center of the oven and make sure there is no rack above it so that nothing interferes with the rising.

Prep Time: 20 minutes

Baking Time: 30 minutes

Serves: 4

2 tablespoons virgin olive oil

3 cups wild mushrooms, diced (12 ounces stemmed)

½ cup minced shallots

1 teaspoon dried fines herbes

¼ teaspoon sea salt

¼ teaspoon ground black pepper

¼ cup white wine

2 tablespoons diced Italian parsley

⅔ cup grated Gruyère cheese

8 large organic-fed, cage-free eggs, separated

Garnish

1 tablespoon chopped Italian parsley

2 tablespoons grated Parmesan cheese

2 tablespoons grated Gruyère cheese

2 tablespoons almond slivers

Preheat oven to 400°F. Lightly butter soufflé dish (9 inches wide by 5 inches high) or 1½-quart baking dish.

Heat sauté pan to medium-high, add oil, then mushrooms, shallots, fines herbes, salt, and black pepper. Sauté, stirring occasionally, until mushrooms are soft and tender, 4–5 minutes; add white wine to deglaze the pan and stir 30 seconds. Stir in parsley, remove from heat, and stir in ⅔ cup grated Gruyère.

In a large bowl, beat egg yolks together. Add mushroom mixture to yolks.

In a separate bowl, beat egg whites until stiff. Then gently fold into mushroom mixture (don't overmix or the soufflé won't rise) and pour into prepared soufflé or baking dish. Top with parsley, remaining cheeses, and almond slivers. Bake at 400°F for 30–35 minutes, until a skewer comes out clean. Serve immediately.

Nutrient Content Per Serving

Calories: 322	Protein: 21 grams
Fiber: 1 gram	Carbs: 5.5 grams
Sodium: 560 milligrams	Fat: 23 grams

Side Dishes

Purple Potatoes with Garlic, Herbs, and Parsley

This is a terrific side dish for many menus.

Prep Time: 10 minutes
Cooking Time: 6-8 minutes
Serves: 4

1½ pounds purple potatoes, quartered
2 tablespoons extra-virgin olive oil
1 teaspoon dried Italian herbs
1 medium garlic clove, diced
½ cup chopped Italian parsley (save a few tablespoons
for a garnish)

Bring 3 quarts water and 1 teaspoon salt to a boil, add potatoes and boil 6-8 minutes, or until they can be pierced with a fork. Do not overcook.

Meanwhile, heat olive oil in a pan over medium-low heat and add herbs, garlic, and parsley. Sauté briefly, watching closely so garlic does not brown. Remove from heat.

When potatoes are done, drain and transfer to a serving bowl. Add garlic and herb mixture and gently toss before serving.

Nutrient Content Per Serving

Calories: 197	Protein: 3.8 grams
Fiber: 4 grams	Carbs: 3 grams
Sodium: 15 milligrams	Fat: 7.2 grams

When it comes to potatoes, always go for color. Purple potatoes, for instance, have far more nutrients and a much lower glycemic load than white potatoes. Colorful potatoes are filled with healthy carotenoids (and some flavonoids) that white potatoes don't have.

Sautéed Kale with Garlic and Lemon

This simple side dish can be prepared quickly.

Prep and Cooking Time: 7-10 minutes

Serves: 2

1 tablespoon almond oil (or any nut oil)

4 cups chopped kale

2 slices lemon, diced

¼ teaspoon sea salt

¼ teaspoon ground black pepper

2 medium garlic cloves, diced

Heat a sauté pan to medium heat. Add oil, then kale, lemon, salt, and pepper. Heat 2 minutes, stirring occasionally. Add garlic and cook another 2 minutes, stirring occasionally. Serve immediately.

Nutrient Content Per Serving

Calories: 132	Protein: 4.6 grams
Fiber: 3 grams	Carbs: 14.5 grams
Sodium: 353 milligrams	Fat: 8 grams

Kale is truly a superstar—being a great source of vitamin K, fiber, potassium, calcium, and many more nutrients! Its "superfood" label is well-deserved.

Brussels Sprouts
with Smart Lemon-Butter Sauce

Smart Lemon-Butter Sauce is great with many vegetables and a delicious way to add some smart fat and extra nutrients to a traditional butter sauce. Here it is with Brussels sprouts.

Prep Time: 10 minutes

Cooking Time: 8-10 minutes

Serves: 2

2 pounds Brussels sprouts, trimmed and halved

1 tablespoon salted organic butter

1 tablespoon virgin olive oil

½ tablespoon grated organic lemon rind

½ tablespoon lemon juice

1 medium garlic clove, minced

¼ teaspoon dried thyme

Steam Brussels sprout halves 6-8 minutes, until tender but still al dente.

Combine butter, oil, lemon rind and juice, garlic, and thyme. Cook briefly over medium heat, taking care not to brown the garlic. Remove from heat. Toss with Brussels sprouts and serve.

Nutrient Content Per Serving

Calories: 308	Protein: 15.5 grams
Fiber: 17 grams	Carbs: 41 grams
Sodium: 155 milligrams	Fat: 14 grams

Sautéed Swiss Chard with Garlic and Italian Herbs

Another easy, delicious side dish that you can prepare in just minutes.

Prep and Cooking Time: 7-10 minutes

Serves: 2

1 tablespoon virgin olive oil

4 cups chopped Swiss chard

¼ teaspoon sea salt

¼ teaspoon ground black pepper

1 teaspoon dried Italian herbs

4 medium garlic cloves, minced

Heat a sauté pan to medium heat; add oil, Swiss chard, salt, pepper, herbs, and garlic, stirring occasionally 3-4 minutes until Swiss chard has wilted. Remove from heat and serve.

Nutrient Content Per Serving

Calories: 83	Protein: 2 grams
Fiber: 1.5 grams	Carbs: 5 grams
Sodium: 449 milligrams	Fat: 7 grams

Wild Rice and Quinoa
with Kale and Slivered Almonds

This flavor-packed combo is loaded with nutrients. Add any type of bean and a veggie of your choice and this becomes a terrific lunch, side dish, or even light dinner.

Prep Time: 30 minutes
Simmering Time: 20 minutes
Serves: 4

½ cup wild rice, rinsed and drained

½ cup quinoa, rinsed and drained

3 cups low-sodium organic vegetable or chicken broth

1½ tablespoons pecan oil (or almond oil)

½ medium sweet onion, cut into 1- to 2-inch slivers

½ teaspoon sea salt

¼ teaspoon ground black pepper

1 teaspoon dried Italian herbs

½ teaspoon ground paprika

4 cups chopped kale (4-6 large leaves)

15-ounce can garbanzo beans, rinsed and drained

½ cup slivered or sliced almonds (or chopped pecans)

½ cup grated Parmesan cheese

Combine rinsed and drained wild rice with 2 cups broth in a medium saucepan, bring to a boil, then cover and reduce to medium-low heat for 45-55 minutes until rice is chewy and some of the grains have burst open. Drain the rice in a strainer and set aside.

Meanwhile, combine rinsed and drained quinoa with remaining 1 cup broth in a medium saucepan. Bring to a boil, then reduce to a simmer for 10-15 minutes. When quinoa is tender and the pearly white tips burst from the grain, it is done; be careful not to overcook. Drain and set aside.

Next, heat a sauté pan to medium-high heat, add oil, then onion, salt, black pepper, and Italian herbs. Cook about 3 minutes, until onion is translucent. Add paprika and kale; reduce heat to medium and cook another 2 minutes until kale has softened. Add beans, cover, and reduce heat to low for 2 minutes, stirring occasionally.

In a sauté pan, heat almonds over medium-low heat 1–2 minutes until toasted but not browned. Mix wild rice with quinoa, then stir in the vegetable mixture and slivered almonds. Garnish with Parmesan cheese. Serve hot or cold.

Nutrient Content Per Serving

Calories: 457	Protein: 19.5 grams
Fiber: 12 grams	Carbs: 62 grams
Sodium: 747 milligrams	Fat: 17.7 grams

Desserts

Cherry-Ricotta Swirl

You'll look forward to eating this calcium-rich dessert. You can make it in advance and refrigerate for a day or two.

Prep Time: 10 minutes (with food processor or blender)
Serves: 2

- **2 cups frozen cherries (unsweetened)**
- **1 cup organic ricotta cheese (part-skim or full-fat)**
- **1 grated organic lemon rind**
- **1 tablespoon lemon juice**
- **1 pinch sea salt**
- **2 tablespoons port wine**
- **1 tablespoon maple syrup or honey (optional)**
- **2 tablespoons slivered almonds (for garnish)**

Blend ingredients in food processor or blender until smooth. If you like some cherry chunks, save a few cherries to add at the very end. Garnish with slivered almonds and serve.

Nutrient Content Per Serving

Calories: 339	Protein: 16.5 grams
Fiber: 4 grams	Carbs: 37 grams
Sodium: 195 milligrams	Fat: 13 grams

Pumpkin Pudding

Pumpkin has a very low glycemic load, and the eggs and milk lower it more, so even with the maple syrup, this remains a medium-GL dish and worth a splurge for a special occasion. Move over, pumpkin pie–this tastes even better!

Prep Time: 10 minutes (with food processor or blender)
Baking Time: 60 minutes
Serves: 6

15 ounces canned pumpkin purée, unsweetened
½ cup maple syrup
¼ teaspoon sea salt
1 teaspoon ground cinnamon
1 tablespoon minced candied gingerroot
¼ teaspoon ground cloves
Dash of ground cayenne pepper
6 large organic-fed, cage-free eggs
1 cup organic whole milk
½ cup organic cream, whipped (optional)

Preheat oven to 400°F. Lightly butter pie pan or baking dish. Combine ingredients in blender or food processor and purée. Pour into pan and bake 10 minutes, then reduce heat to 350°F for 50 minutes. Remove from oven, let cool, then refrigerate 2-3 hours to solidify. Serve with a garnish of whipped cream.

Nutrient Content Per Serving

Calories: 285	Protein: 9.2 grams
Fiber: 3 grams	Carbs: 26 grams
Sodium: 215 milligrams	Fat: 8 grams

Dark Chocolate Drizzle

Fruit is good by itself but even better with this special drizzle.
Serves: 2

2 ounces dark chocolate
1 tablespoon organic butter

2 cups fruit (apple, orange, pitted cherries, strawberries), cut in bite-size pieces

2 tablespoons chopped nuts of your choice

In double boiler, melt chocolate, then add butter and stir together; alternatively, melt slowly together in a glass bowl in microwave. Spread fruit pieces over a plate and drizzle with chocolate; sprinkle with chopped nuts. Serve immediately or chill and save for later.

Nutrient Content Per Serving

Calories: 260	Protein: 3.5 grams
Fiber: 5 grams	Carbs: 33 grams
Sodium: 2 milligrams	Fat: 16 grams

Fruit Salad with Mint, Lemon Rind, and Greek Yogurt

This simple, delicious fruit salad is in the dessert section, but it can also be a great breakfast or snack. Use organic yogurt–full-fat, reduced-fat, or skim, whatever you prefer. Use any fruit you like. Steven picks two or three from berries, apples, pears, kiwi, grapes, melons, and pomegranate seeds.

Prep Time: 5-10 minutes
Serves: 2

1 cup organic, plain Greek yogurt

2 cups mixed fruit

1 tablespoon grated organic lemon rind

1 tablespoon lemon juice

¼ cup fresh mint, chopped

2 tablespoons walnuts or pistachios, chopped and toasted

Combine all ingredients in a serving bowl. Top with nuts.

Nutrient Content Per Serving

Calories: 193	Protein: 6.8 grams
Fiber: 4.2 grams	Carbs: 26.5 grams
Sodium: 155 milligrams	Fat: 8 grams

Fruit and Nut Crumble

You can vary the fruit and nuts with what you find in your pantry, and the result will always be satisfying!

Prep Time: 15 minutes
Baking Time: 15 minutes
Serves: 6

1 teaspoon almond oil (for pie pan)
2 tablespoons almond butter
2 tablespoons organic salted butter
¼ cup maple syrup
2 medium pears, cut into ½-inch cubes
2 medium apples, cut into ½-inch cubes
⅛ teaspoon salt
½ teaspoon ground cinnamon
½ medium organic orange, juiced and rind grated
¼ cup port wine
1 cup fresh raspberries or blackberries
¼ cup rolled oats
½ cup almond slivers
½ cup chopped pecans
½ cup organic cream, whipped (optional)

Preheat oven to 375°F. Lightly oil pie pan with almond oil.

Heat a medium saucepan over medium heat and add almond butter, butter, maple syrup, pears, apples, salt, and cinnamon; bring to bubbling, then add orange juice and rind. Reduce heat to low and add port wine. Simmer 5 minutes; add berries and remove from heat.

Meanwhile, heat a sauté pan to medium-low heat, toast oats 3–4 minutes, stirring occasionally, until slightly golden; add almonds and pecans, toast another 2 minutes until warm, then remove from heat.

Pour fruit mixture into pie pan; sprinkle oats and nuts on top. Bake 15 minutes and serve. If desired, top each serving with a dollop of whipped cream.

Nutrient Content Per Serving

Calories: 313	Protein: 5 grams
Fiber: 7 grams	Carbs: 33 grams
Sodium: 33 milligrams	Fat: 19 grams

References

The following references are provided for readers interested in more information and exploration.

Chapter 1. A High-Fat Diet for a Low-Fat Body

Astrup A et al. Atkins and other low-carbohydrate diets: Hoax or an effective tool for weight loss? *Lancet*. 2004; 364: 897–99.

Aude YW et al. The National Cholesterol Education Program diet vs. a diet lower in carbohydrates and higher in protein and monounsaturated fat: A randomized trial. *Arch Intern Med*. 2004; 164(19): 2141–46.

Brehm BJ et al. A randomized trial comparing a very low carbohydrate diet and a calorie-restricted low fat diet on body weight and cardiovascular risk factors in healthy women. *J Clin Endocrinol Metab*. 2003; 88: 1617–23.

Foster GD et al. Randomized trial of a low-carb diet for obesity. *N Engl J Med*. 2003; 348: 2082–90.

Kolasa KM, Deen D, eds., for the Society of Teachers of Family Medicine Group on Nutrition. *Physician's Curriculum in Clinical Nutrition: Primary Care*. 2nd ed. (Society of Teachers of Family Medicine, 2005).

Masley SC. Dietary therapy for preventing and treating coronary artery disease. *Am Fam Physician*. 1998; 57: 1299–1306.

———. Enhancing dietary adherence. *Permanente Forum*. September 1998.

———. Group visits for chronic illness care. *Fam Pract Manag*. 2006; 13: 21–22.

———. Improving dietary compliance, how can we do a better job? *Group Health Forum*. October 1996.

———. "Measuring Physical Fitness." Chapter 16 in Evans CH, White RD, eds. *Exercise Testing for Primary Care and Sports Medicine* (Springer, 2009).

———. Top five nutritional deficiencies, and how to correct them. *Cortlandt Forum*. October/November 2008.

Masley SC et al. Aerobic exercise enhances cognitive flexibility. *J Clinical Psychol*. 2009; 16: 186–93.

———. Blood pressure as a predictor of CVD events in the elderly: The William E. Hale research program. *J Hum Hypertens*. 2006; 20(6): 392–97.

———. Cardiovascular biomarkers and carotid IMT scores as predictors of cognitive function. *J Am Coll Nutr*. 2014; 33(1): 63–69.

————. Effect of mercury levels and seafood intake on cognitive function in middle-aged adults. *Int Med.* 2012; 11: 32–40.

————. Efficacy of exercise and diet to modify markers of fitness and wellness. *Altern Ther Health Med.* 2008; 14: 24–29.

————. Emerging lifestyle factors predict carotid intimal media thickness scores. *Circulation.* 2014; 129: AP433.

————. Emerging risk factors as predictors of carotid intima media thickness scores. *J Am Coll Nutr.* 201534(2):100–7.

————. Group office visits change dietary habits of patients with coronary artery disease: The dietary intervention and evaluation trial (D.I.E.T.). *J Fam Pract.* 2001; 50(3): 235–39.

————. High-fiber, low-saturated fat diet combined with exercise enhances VO2max and lipid profiles. *Circulation.* 2006; 113: e380 (abstract).

————. Impact of an exercise and dietary program on weight loss. *J Am Coll Nutr.* 2005; 24: 431 (abstract).

————. Planning group visits for high-risk patients. *Fam Pract Manag.* 2000: 7(6): 33–36.

Samaha FF et al. A low-carb as compared with a low-fat diet in severe obesity. *N Engl J Med.* 2003; 348: 2074–87.

Stern L et al. The effects of low-carb versus conventional weight loss diets in severely obese adults: One-year follow up of a randomized trial. *Ann Intern Med.* 2004; 140: 778–85.

Theobold M, Masley SC. *A Guide to Group Visits for Chronic Condition Affected by Overweight and Obesity.* American Academy of Family Physicians, Americans in Motion (AIM) Monograph, 2008.

————. *A Guide to Tobacco Cessation Group Visits. Ask and Act, a Tobacco Cessation Program.* American Academy of Family Physicians Monograph, 2007.

Willi SM et al. The effects of a high-protein, low-fat ketogenic diet on adolescents with morbid obesity: Body composition, blood chemistries, and sleep abnormalities. *Pediatrics.* 1998; 101: 61–67.

Chapter 2. Why the Smart Fat Solution Will Make You Lean and Healthy

Afshin A et al. Consumption of nuts and legumes and risk of incident ischemic heart disease, stroke, and diabetes: A systematic review and meta-analysis. *Am J Clin Nutr.* 2014; 100: 278–88.

Akduman B et al. Effect of statins on serum prostate-specific antigen levels. *Urology.* 2010; 76: 1048–51.

Azadbakht L et al. The dietary approaches to stop hypertension eating plan affects C-reactive protein, coagulation abnormalities, and hepatic function tests among type 2 diabetic patients. *J Nutr* 2011; 141: 1083–88.

Bazzano LA et al. Effects of low-carb and low-fat diets. *Ann Intern Med.* 2014; 161: 309–18.

Berthold HK et al. Effect of a garlic oil preparation on serum lipoproteins and cholesterol metabolism (deodorized garlic). *JAMA.* 1998; 279: 1900–1902.

Buil-Cosiales P et al. Fiber intake and all-cause mortality in the Prevencion con Dieta Mediterranea (PREDIMED) study. *Am J Clin Nutr.* 2014; 100: 1498–507.

Chait A, Kim F. Saturated fatty acids and inflammation: Who pays the toll? *Arterioscler Thromb Vasc Biol.* 2010; 30: 692–93.

Chandalia M et al. Beneficial effects of high dietary fiber intake in patients with type 2 diabetes mellitus. *N Engl J Med.* 2000; 342: 1392–98.

Chowdhury R et al. Association of dietary, circulating, and supplement fatty acids with coronary risk: A systematic review and meta-analysis. *Ann Intern Med.* 2014; 160(6): 398–406.

Corona G. The effect of statin therapy on testosterone levels in subjects consulting for erectile dysfunction. *J Sex Med.* 2010; 7: 1547–56.

Dansinger ML et al. Comparison of the Atkins, Ornish, Weight Watchers, and Zone diets for weight loss and heart disease risk reduction: A randomized trial. *JAMA.* 2005; 293(1): 43–53.

Deopurkar R et al. Differential effects of cream, glucose, and orange juice on inflammation, endotoxin, and the expression of toll-like receptor–4 and suppressor of cytokine signaling–3. *Diabetes Care.* 2010; 33: 991–97.

Dobs A et al. Effects of high-dose simvastatin on adrenal and gonadal steroidogenesis in men with hypercholesterolemia. *Metabolism.* 2000; 29: 1234–38.

Donnelly JE et al. Effects of a 16-month randomized controlled exercise trial on body weight and composition in young, overweight, men and women. *Arch Intern Med.* 2003; 163: 1343–50.

Estruch R et al. Primary prevention of cardiovascular disease with a Mediterranean diet. *N Engl J Med.* 2013; 368: 1279–90.

Forsythe CE et al. Limited effect of dietary saturated fat on plasma saturated fat in the context of a low carbohydrate diet. *Lipids.* 2010; 45: 947–62.

Foster GD et al. A randomized trial of the effects of an almond-enriched, hypocaloric diet in the treatment of obesity. *Am J Clin Nutr.* 2012; 96(2): 249–54.

Funaki M. Saturated fatty acids and insulin resistance. *J Med Invest.* 2009; 56: 88–92.

Grosso G et al. Nut consumption on all-cause cardiovascular, and cancer mortality risk: A systematic review and meta-analysis of epidemiologic studies. *Am J Clin Nutr.* 2015; 101: 783–93.

Halton TL, Hu FB. The effects of high protein diets on thermogensis, satiety, and weight loss. *J Am Coll Nutr.* 2004; 23: 373–83.

Harcombe Z et al. Evidence from randomized controlled trials did not support the introduction of dietary fat guidelines in 1977 and 1983: A systemic review and meta-analysis. *Open Heart.* 2015; 2: e000196. doi:10.1136/openhrt–2014–000196.

Harman D. Free radical theory of aging. *Mutat Res.* 1992; 275(3–6): 257–66.

Himaya A et al. Satiety power of dietary fat: A new appraisal. *Am J Clin Nutr.* 1997; 65(5): 1410–18.

Holt SHA et al. A satiety index of common foods. *Eur J Clin Nutr.* 1995; 49: 675–90.

Hshieh TT et al. Nut consumption and risk of mortality in the Physicians' Health Study. *Am J Clin Nutr.* 2015; 101: 407–12.

Hu FB. The Mediterranean diet and mortality: Olive oil and beyond. *N Engl J Med.* 2003; 108: 1554–59.

Hu FB et al. Frequent nut consumption and risk of coronary heart disease in women. *BMJ.* 1998; 17: 1341–45.

Kris-Etherton PM et al. The effects of nuts on coronary heart disease risk. *Nutr Rev.* 2001; 59: 103–11.

———. High-monounsaturated fatty acid diets lower both plasma cholesterol and triacylglycerol concentrations. *Am J Clin Nutr.* 1999; 70: 1009–15.

Kuipers RS et al. Saturated fat, carbohydrates, and cardiovascular disease. *J Med.* 2011; 69: 372–78.

Larsen LF et al. Are olive oil diets antithrombotic? Diets enriched with olive, rapeseed, or sunflower oil affect postprandial factor VII differently. *Am J Clin Nutr.* 1999; 70: 976–82.

Lawrence GD. Dietary fats and health: Dietary recommendations in the context of scientific evidence. *Adv Nutr.* 2013; 4: 294–302.

Lopez-Garcia E et al. Consumption of trans fatty acids is related to plasma biomarkers of inflammation and endothelial dysfunction. *J Nutr.* 2005; 135: 562–66.

Messina M. Soy foods, isoflavones, and the health of postmenopausal women. *Am J Clin Nutr.* 2014; 100(suppl): 423S–30S.

Muller H et al. A diet rich in coconut oil reduces diurnal postprandial variations in circulating tissue plasminogen activator antigen and fasting lipoprotein (a) compared with a diet rich in unsaturated fat in women. *J Nutr.* 2003; 133: 3422–27.

Nielsen SJ, Popkin BM. Patterns and trends in food portion sizes, 1977–1998. *JAMA.* 2003; 289: 450–53.

Olshansky SJ et al. A potential decline in life expectancy in the US in the 21st century. *N Engl J Med.* 2005; 352: 1138–45.

Rajaram S. Health benefits of plant-derived alpha-linolenic acid. *Am J Clin Nutr.* 2014; 100(suppl): 443S–48S.

Renaud S et al. Cretan Mediterranean diet for prevention of coronary heart disease. *Am J Clin Nutr.* 1995; 61: 1360S–67S.

Ridker PM et al. C-reactive protein and other markers of inflammation in the prediction of cardiovascular disease in women. *N Engl J Med.* 2000; 342: 836–43.

Rolls BJ et al. What can intervention studies tell us about the relationship between fruit and vegetable consumption and weight management? *Nutr Rev.* 2004; 62: 1–17.

Sabate J et al. Effects of walnuts on serum lipid levels and blood pressure in men. *N Engl J Med.* 1993; 328: 603–7.

Sanders TAB. Plant compared with marine n–3 fatty acid effects on cardiovascular risk factors and outcomes: What is the verdict? *Am J Clin Nutr.* 2014; 100(suppl): 453S–58S.

Schwartz EA et al. Nutrient modification and the innate immune response: A novel mechanism by which saturated fatty acids greatly amplify monocyte inflammation. *Arterioscler Thromb Vasc Biol.* 2010; 30(4): 802–8.

Sesso HD et al. C-reactive protein and the risk of developing hypertension. *JAMA.* 2003; 290: 2945–51.

Silagy CA, Neil HA. A meta-analysis of the effect of garlic on blood pressure. *J Hypertens.* 1994; 12: 463–68.

Simopoulos AP, De Meester F, eds. *A Balanced Omega–6/Omega–3 Fatty Acid Ratio, Cholesterol and Coronary Heart Disease* (Karger, 2008).

Skender ML et al. Comparison of 2-year weight loss trends in behavioral treatments of obesity: Diet, exercise, and combination interventions. *J Am Diet Assoc.* 1996; 96: 342–46.

Smith SC. Need for a paradigm shift: The importance of risk factor reduction therapy in treating patients with cardiovascular disease. *Am J Cardiol.* 1998; 82: 10–13.

Solà R et al. Cocoa, hazelnuts, sterols, and soluble fiber cream reduce lipids and inflammation biomarkers in hypertensive patients. *PLoS ONE.* 2012; 7(2): e31103. doi: 10.1371/journal .pone.0031103.

Spiller GA et al. Effects of plant-based diets high in raw or roasted almonds or almond butter on serum lipoproteins in humans. *J Am Coll Nutr.* 2003; 22: 195–200.

Srivastava KC et al. Effects of a garlic-derived principle on aggregation and arachidonic acid metabolism in human blood platelets. *Prostaglandins Leukot Essent Fatty Acids.* 1993; 49: 587–95.

Steiner M et al. A double-blind crossover study in moderately hypercholesterolemic men that compared the effect of aged garlic extract and placebo administration on blood lipids. *Am J Clin Nutr.* 1996; 64: 866–70.

St-Onge M-P. Dietary fats, teas, dairy and nuts: Potential functional foods for weight control? *Am J Clin Nutr.* 2005; 81: 7–15.

Streppel MT et al. Dietary fiber and blood pressure. *Arch Intern Med.* 2005; 165: 150–56.

Tan SY et al. A review of the effects of nuts on appetite, food intake, metabolism, and body weight. *Am J Clin Nutr.* 2014; 100(suppl): 412S–22S.

Tattelman E. Health effects of garlic. *Am Fam Physician*. 2005; 72: 103–6.

U.S. Department of Health and Human Services, Agency for Healthcare Research and Quality. "Health effects of omega–3 fatty acids on cardiovascular risk factors and intermediate markers of cardiovascular disease." March 2004. http://archive.ahrq.gov/clinic/tp/o3cardrisktp.htm.

Van de Laar RJJ et al. Lower lifetime dietary fiber intake is associated with carotid artery stiffness. *Am J Clin Nutr*. 2012; 96: 14–23.

Willett WC. Dietary fat and obesity: An unconvincing relation. *Am J Clin Nutr*. 1998; 68: 1149–50.

Wing RR, Hill JO. Successful weight loss maintenance. *Ann Rev Nutr*. 2001; 21: 323–41.

Yakoob MY et al. Circulating biomarkers of dairy fat and risk of incident stroke in US men and women in 2 large prospective cohorts. *Am J Clin Nutr*. 2014; 100: 1437–47.

Yaqoob P et al. Effect of olive oil on immune function in middle-aged men. *Am J Clin Nutr*. 1998; 67: 129–35.

Yusuf S et al. Effect of potentially modifiable risk factors associated with myocardial infarction in 52 countries (the INTERHEART study). *Lancet*. 2004; 364: 937–52.

Zhao G et al. Dietary alpha-linolenic acid inhibits proinflammatory cytokine production by peripheral blood mononuclear cells in hypercholesterolemic subjects. *Am J Clin Nutr*. 2007; 85: 385–91.

Chapter 3. What *Not* to Eat

Bellavia A et al. Differences in survival associated with processed and with nonprocessed red meat consumption. *Am J Clin Nutr*. 2014; 100: 924–29.

Byers T. Hardened fats, hardened arteries? *N Engl J Med*. 1997; 337: 1544–45.

Daley, CA et al. A review of fatty acid profiles and antioxidant content in grass-fed and grain-fed beef. *Nutrition Journal* 2010; 9:10.

DiNicolantonio JJ et al. The wrong white crystals: Not salt but sugar as aetiological in hypertension and cardiometabolic disease. *Open Heart*. 2014; 1e000167. doi: 10.1136/openhrt–2014–000167.

Fuller NR et al. The effect of a high-egg diet on cardiovascular risk factors in people with type 2 diabetes: The Diabetes and Egg (DIABEGG) study. *Am J Clin Nutr*. 2015; 101: 705–13.

Judd JT et al. Effects of margarine compared with those of butter on blood lipid profiles related to cardiovascular disease risk factors in normolipemic adults fed controlled diets. *Am J Clin Nutr*. 1998; 68: 768–77.

King IB et al. Serum trans-fatty acids are associated with risk of prostate cancer in beta-carotene and retinol efficacy trial. *Cancer Epidemiol Biomarkers Prev*. 2005; 14: 988–92.

Kris-Etherton PM, Nicolosi RJ. Trans fatty acids and coronary heart disease risk: Report of the expert panel on trans fatty acids and coronary heart disease. *Am J Clin Nutr*. 1995; 62(3): 655S–708S.

Pesatori AC et al. Cancer incidence in the population exposed to dioxin after the Seveso accident. *Environ Health*. 2009; 8: 39.

Raloff J. "Hormones: Here's the Beef." Science News Online. http://www.phschool.com/science/science_news/articles/hormones_beef.html.

Ramsden CE et al. Lowering dietary linoleic acid reduces bioactive oxidized linoleic acid metabolites in humans. *Prostaglandins Leukot Essent Fatty Acids*. 2012; 87(4–5): 135–41.

Ramsden CE et al. Use of dietary linoleic acid for secondary prevention of coronary heart disease and death: Evaluation of recovered data from the Sydney Diet Heart Study and updated meta-analysis. *BMJ*. 2013; 346: e8707.

Simopoulos AP. The importance of the ratio of omega–6/omega–3 fatty acids. *Biomed Pharmacother.* 2002; 56: 365–79.

Vega CP. "Is Sugar the Real Culprit Behind Hypertension?" Medscape. http://www.medscape.org/viewarticle/837050.

White SS, Birnbaum LS. An overview of the effects of dioxins and dioxin-like compounds on vertebrates, as documented in human and ecological epidemiology. *J Environ Sci Health C Environ Carcinog Ecotoxicol Rev.* 2009 Oct; 27(4): 197–211.

Chapter 4. Unlearn What You Know About Food

"About Metabolic Syndrome." American Heart Association. http://www.heart.org/HEARTORG/Conditions/More/MetabolicSyndrome/About-Metabolic-Syndrome_UCM_301920_Article.jsp.

Albu JB et al. Metabolic changes following a 1-year diet and exercise intervention in patients with type 2 diabetes. *Diabetes.* 2010; 59(3): 627–33.

American Heart Association. "Heart Disease and Stroke Continue to Threaten U.S. Health: American Heart Association Annual Statistical Update." http://newsroom.heart.org/news/heart-disease-and-stroke-continue-to-threaten-u-s-health.

Anderson GH, Woodend D. Effect of glycemic carbohydrates on short-term satiety and food intake. *Nutr Rev.* 2003; 61: S17–S26.

Aude YW et al. The National Cholesterol Education Program diet vs. a diet lower in carbohydrates and higher in protein and monounsaturated fat: A randomized trial. *Arch Intern Med.* 2004; 164(19): 2141–46.

Aune D et al. Carbohydrates, glycemic index, glycemic load, and colorectal cancer risk. *Cancer Causes Control.* 2012; 23: 521–35.

Brand-Miller JC et al. Glycemic index and obesity. *Am J Clin Nutr.* 2002; 76: 281S–85S.

———. Glycemic load and chronic disease. *Nutr Rev.* 2003; 61: S49–S55.

———. *The New Glucose Revolution* (Marlowe, 2003).

Bray GA. How bad is fructose? *Am J Clin Nutr.* 2007; 86: 895–96.

Bruce WR et al. Mechanisms linking diet and colorectal cancer. *Nutr Cancer.* 2000; 37: 19–26.

Chowdhury R et al. Association of dietary, circulating, and supplement fatty acids with coronary risk: A systematic review and meta-analysis. *Ann Intern Med.* 2014; 160(6): 398–406.

Dong JY, Qin LQ. Dietary glycemic index, glycemic load, and risk of breast cancer. *Breast Cancer Res Treat.* 2011; 126: 287–94.

Eckel RH et al. The metabolic syndrome. *Lancet.* 2005; 365: 1415–28.

Frost G. Glycaemic index as a determinant of serum HDL-cholesterol concentration. *Lancet.* 1999; 353: 1045–48.

Giacco R et al. Long-term dietary treatment with increased amounts of fibre-rich low-glycemic index natural foods improves blood glucose control and reduces the number of hypoglycemic events in type 1 diabetic patients. *Diabetes Care.* 2000; 23: 1461–66.

Grundy SM. Inflammation, hypertension, and the metabolic syndrome. *JAMA.* 2003; 290: 3000–3002.

Grundy SM et al. AHA/NHLBI Scientific Statement: Diagnosis and management of the metabolic syndrome. *Circulation.* 2005; 112: 2735–52.

Henry FI et al. The metabolic syndrome, cardiopulmonary fitness, and subcutaneous trunk fat as independent determinants of arterial stiffness: The Amsterdam Growth and Health Longitudinal Study. *Arch Intern Med.* 2005; 165: 875–82.

Hu J et al. Glycemic index, glycemic load and cancer risk. *Ann Oncol.* 2013; 24: 245–51.

"IDF Worldwide Definition of the Metabolic Syndrome." International Diabetes Federation. http://www.idf.org/metabolic-syndrome.

Jessup A et al. Metabolic syndrome: Look for it in children and adolescents, too! *Clin Diabetes.* 2005; 23: 26–32.

Johnson RJ et al. Potential role of sugar (fructose) in the epidemic of hypertension, obesity and the metabolic syndrome, diabetes, kidney disease, and cardiovascular disease. *Am J Clin Nutr.* 2007; 86(4): 899–906.

Kumari M et al. Minireview: Mechanisms by which the metabolic syndrome and diabetes impair memory. *J Gerontol A Biol Sci Med Sci.* 2000; 55(5): B228–32.

Laukkanen JA et al. Metabolic syndrome and the risk of prostate cancer in Finnish men: A population based study. *Cancer Epidemiol Biomarkers Prev.* 2004; 13: 1646–50.

Mancini MC. Metabolic syndrome in children and adolescents: Criteria for diagnosis. *Diabetol Metab Syndr.* 2009; 1: 20.

McKeown NM et al. Carbohydrate nutrition, insulin resistance, and the prevalence of the metabolic syndrome in the Framingham Offspring Cohort. *Diabetes Care.* 2004; 27: 538–46.

Ness KK et al. Prevalence of the metabolic syndrome in relation to self-reported cancer history. *Ann Epidemiol.* 2005; 15: 202–6.

Orchard TJ et al. The effect of Metformin and intensive lifestyle intervention on the metabolic syndrome: The Diabetes Prevention Program randomized trial. *Ann Intern Med.* 2005; 142: 611–19.

Reaven GM. Diet and Syndrome X. *Curr Atheroscler Rep.* 2000; 2: 503–7.

———. Metabolic syndrome: Pathophysiology and implications for management of cardiovascular disease. *Circulation.* 2002; 106: 286–88.

Salmeron J et al. Dietary fiber, glycemic load, and risk of non-insulin-dependent diabetes in women. *JAMA.* 1997; 277: 472–77.

Salonen JT et al. HDL, HDL2, and HDL3 subfractions, and the risk of acute myocardial infarction: A prospective population study in eastern Finnish men. *Circulation.* 1991; 84: 129–39.

Samaha FF et al. A low-carbohydrate as compared with a low-fat diet in severe obesity. *N Engl J Med.* 2003; 348: 2074–81.

Saris WHM. Glycemic carbohydrate and body weight regulation. *Nutr Rev.* 2003; 61: S10–S16.

Siri-Tarino PW et al. Meta-analysis of prospective cohort studies evaluating the association of saturated fat with cardiovascular disease. *Am J Clin Nutr.* 2010; 91(3): 535–46.

Sondike SB et al. Effects of a low-carbohydrate diet on weight loss and cardiovascular risk factor in overweight adolescents. *J Pediatrics.* 2003; 142(3): 253–58.

Spies C et al. Association of metabolic syndrome with exercise capacity and heart rate recovery in patients with coronary heart disease in the heart and soul study. *Am J Cardiol.* 2005; 95: 1175–79.

Staff of the Select Committee on Nutrition and Human Needs. "Dietary Goals for the United States," presented to the U.S. Senate, 95th Congress, 1st Sess., February 1977 (USGPO, 1977).

U.S. Department of Agriculture. "Profiling Food Consumption in America." Chapter 2 in *Agriculture Fact Book 2001–2002* (USGPO, 2003), 13–21. http://www.usda.gov/factbook/2002factbook.pdf.

Volek JS et al. Carbohydrate restriction has a more favorable impact on the metabolic syndrome than a low fat diet. *Lipids.* 2009; 44(4): 297–309.

Willett W et al. Glycemic index, glycemic load, and risk of type 2 diabetes. *Am J Clin Nutr.* 2002; 76: 274S–80S.

Wolever TMS. The glycemic index. *World Rev Nutr Diet.* 1990; 62: 120–85.

Chapter 5. The Smart Fat Solution

Baer DJ et al. Whey protein but not soy protein supplementation alters body weight and composition in free-living overweight and obese adults. *J Nutr.* 2011; 141(8): 1489–94.

Claesson AL et al. Two weeks of overfeeding with candy, but not peanuts, increases insulin levels and body weight. Only peanuts raise BMR. *Clin Lab Invest.* 2009; 69(5): 598–605.

Coker RH et al. Whey protein and essential amino acids promote the reduction of adipose tissue and increased muscle protein synthesis during caloric restriction–induced weight loss in elderly, obese individuals. *Nutr J.* 2012; 11: 105.

Cruz-Neto AP, Bozinovic F. The relationship between diet quality and basal metabolic rate in endotherms: Insights from intraspecific analysis. *Physiol Biochem Zool.* 2004; 77(6): 877–89.

Fontvieille AM et al. Twenty-four-hour energy expenditure in Pima Indians with type 2 (non-insulin-dependent) diabetes mellitus. *Diabetologia.* 1992; 35(8): 753–59.

Hall WL. Dietary saturated and unsaturated fats as determinants of blood pressure and vascular function. *Nutr Res Rev.* 2009; 22: 18–38.

Halton TL, Hu FB. The effects of high protein diets on thermogenesis, satiety, and weight loss. *J Am Coll Nutr.* 2004; 23: 373–83.

Hermsdorff HH et al. Macronutrient profile affects diet-induced thermogenesis and energy intake [article in Portuguese]. *Arch Latinoam Nutr.* 2007; 57(1): 33–42.

Kantor ED et al. Lifestyle factors and inflammation: Associations by body mass index. *PLoS One.* 2013; 8(7): e67833. doi: 10.1371/journal.pone.0067833.

Nicholls SJ et al. Consumption of saturated fat impairs the anti-inflammatory properties of HDL lipoproteins and endothelial function. *J Am Coll Cardiol.* 2006; 48: 715–20.

Phillips CM et al. Obesity and body fat classification in the metabolic syndrome: Impact on cardiometabolic risk metabotype. *Obesity.* 2013; 21: E154–61.

Sousa GTD et al. Dietary whey protein lessens several risk factors for metabolic diseases: A review. *Lipids Health Dis.* 2012; 11: 67.

Wareham NJ et al. Glucose intolerance and physical inactivity: The relative importance of low habitual energy expenditure and cardiorespiratory fitness. *Am J Epidemiol.* 2000; 152(2): 132–39.

Chapter 6. The Thirty-Day Plan of Smart Fat Meals

Ahmed N et al. Green tea polyphenols and cancer: Biologic mechanisms and practical implications. *Nutr Rev.* 1999; 57: 78–83.

Bell SJ et al. A functional food product for the management of weight. *Crit Rev Food Sci Nutr.* 2002; 42: 163–78.

Geleijnse JM et al. Inverse association of tea and flavonoid intakes with incident myocardial infarction: The Rotterdam Study. *Am J Clin Nutr.* 2002; 75: 880–86.

Ishikawa T et al. Effect of tea flavonoid supplementation on the susceptibility of low-density lipoprotein to oxidative modification. *Am J Clin Nutr.* 1997; 66: 261–66.

Weinreb O et al. Neurological mechanisms of green tea polyphenols in Alzheimer's and Parkinson's diseases. *J Nutr Biochem.* 2004; 15: 506–16.

Chapter 7. The Smart Fat User's Guide

Abou-Donia MB et al. Splenda alters gut microflora and increases intestinal p-glycoprotein and cytochrome p-450 in male rats. *J Toxicol Environ Health A.* 2008; 71(21): 1415–29.

Arkadianos I et al. Improved weight management using genetic information to personalize a calorie controlled diet. *Nutr J.* 2007; 18:6–29.

Astrup A. A changing view on saturated fatty acids and dairy: From enemy to friend. *Am J Clin Nutr.* 2014; 100: 1407–8.

Bagnardi V et al. Alcohol consumption and the risk of cancer: A meta-analysis. *Alcohol Research and Health.* 2001; 25(4): 263–70. http://pubs.niaaa.nih.gov/publications/arh25–4/263–270.pdf.

Beer and spirits, but not wine, raise the risk of upper digestive tract cancer. *BMJ.* 1998; 317: c.

Berger K et al. Light to moderate alcohol consumption and the risk of stroke among US male physicians. *N Engl J Med.* 1999; 341: 1557–64.

Burke LE et al. Self-monitoring in weight loss: A systematic review of the literature. *J Am Diet Assoc.* 2011; 111(1): 92–102.

Bush NC et al. Dietary calcium intake is associated with less gain in intra-abdominal adipose tissue over 1 year. *Obesity (Silver Spring).* 2010; 18(11): 2101–4.

Djousse L, Gaziano JM. Egg consumption and risk of heart failure in the Physicians' Health Study. *Circulation.* 2008; 117: 512–16.

Drehmer M et al. Associations of dairy intake with glycemia and insulinemia independent of obesity in Brazilian adults. *Am J Clin Nutr.* 2015; 101: 775–82.

Dreon DM et al. Change in dietary saturated fat intake is correlated with change in mass of large low-density-lipoprotein particles in men. *Am J Clin Nutr.* 1998; 67(5): 828–36.

Druggan C et al. Protective nutrients and functional foods for the gastrointestinal tract. *Am J Clin Nutr.* 2002; 75: 789–808.

Faridi Z et al. Acute dark chocolate and cocoa ingestion and endothelial function. *Am J Clin Nutr.* 2008; 88: 58–63.

Fernandez ML. Dietary cholesterol provided by eggs and plasma lipoproteins in healthy populations. *Curr Opin Clin Nutr Metab Care.* 2006; 9: 8–12.

Fraga CG. Cocoa, diabetes, and hypertension: Should we eat more chocolate? *Am J Clin Nutr.* 2005; 81: 541–42.

Gilbert JA et al. Milk supplementation facilitates appetite control in obese women during weight loss: A randomised, single-blind, placebo-controlled trial. *Br J Nutr.* 2011; 105(1): 133–43.

Grassi D et al. Short term administration of dark chocolate is followed by a significant increase in insulin sensitivity and a decrease in blood pressure in healthy persons. *Am J Clin Nutr.* 2005; 81: 611–14.

Hainer, V et al. Role of hereditary factors in weight loss and its maintenance. *Physiol Res.* 2008; 57 (suppl 1): S1–15.

Hardy DS et al. Macronutrient intake as a mediator with FTO to increase body mass index. *J Am Coll Nutr.* 2014; 33(4): 256–66.

Harvard T.H. Chan School of Public Health. "Eggs and Heart Disease." *Nutrition Source.* http://www.hsph.harvard.edu/nutritionsource/eggs/#1.

Holahan CJ et al. Wine consumption and 20-year mortality among late life moderate drinkers. *Ann Intern Med.* 2000; 133: 411–19.

Hollis JF et al. Weight loss during the intensive intervention phase of the Weight-Loss Maintenance Trial. *Am J Preventive Med.* 2008; 35(2): 118–26.

Hu FB et al. A prospective study of egg consumption and risk of cardiovascular disease in men and women. *JAMA.* 1999; 281: 1387–94.

Jenkins DJA et al. Effect of legumes as part of a low glycemic index diet on glycemic control and cardiovascular risk factors in type 2 diabetes mellitus. *Arch Intern Med.* 2012; 172: 1653–60.

Jill JO. What do you say when your patients ask whether low-calorie sweeteners help with weight management? *Am J Clin Nutr.* 2014; 100: 739–40.

Josse AR et al. Increased consumption of dairy foods and protein during diet- and exercise-induced weight loss promotes fat mass loss and lean mass gain in overweight and obese premenopausal women. *J Nutr.* 2011; 141(9): 1626–34.

Klatsky AL et al. Alcohol and mortality. *Ann Intern Med.* 1992; 117: 646–54.

Kligler B, Cohrssen A. Probiotics. *Am Fam Physician.* 2008; 78: 1073–78.

Leonard MM, Vasgar B. US perspective on gluten-related diseases. *Clin Experiment Gastroenterol.* 2014; 7: 25–37.

Major GC et al. Calcium plus vitamin D supplementation and fat mass loss in female very low-calcium consumers: Potential link with a calcium-specific appetite control. *Br J Nutr.* 2009; 101(5): 659–63.

———. Supplementation with calcium + vitamin D enhances the beneficial effect of weight loss on plasma lipid and lipoprotein concentrations. *Am J Clin Nutr.* 2007; 85(1): 54–59.

Matroiacovo D et al. Cocoa flavanol consumption improves cognitive function, blood pressure control, and metabolic profile in elderly subjects. *Am J Clin Nutr.* 2015; 101: 538–48.

Matsumoto C et al. Chocolate consumption and risk of diabetes mellitus in the Physicians' Health Study. *Am J Clin Nutr.* 2015; 101: 362–67.

Merino J et al. Is complying with the recommendations of sodium intake beneficial for health in individuals at high cardiovascular risk? Findings from the PREDIMED study. *Am J Clin Nutr.* 2015; 101(3): 440–48.

Messina V. Nutritional and health benefits of dried beans. *Am J Clin Nutr.* 2014; 100(suppl 1): 437S–42S.

Miller PE et al. Low-calorie sweeteners and body weight and composition: A meta-analysis of randomized controlled trials and prospective cohort studies. *Am J Clin Nutr.* 2014; 100: 765–77.

Moreno-Aliaga MJ, et al. Does weight loss prognosis depend on genetic make-up? *Obes Rev* 2004; 6(2): 155–68.

Razquin C et al. A 3-year intervention with a Mediterranean diet modified the association between the rs9939609 gene variant in FTO and body weight changes. *International Journal of Obesity* 2010; 34: 266–72.

Rein D et al. Cocoa inhibits platelet activation and function. *Am J Clin Nutr.* 2000; 72: 30–35.

Rimm EB, Ellison RC. Alcohol in the Mediterranean diet. *Am J Clin Nutr.* 1995; 61: 1378–82.

Rodríguez-Rodríguez E et al. An adequate calcium intake could help achieve weight loss in overweight/obese women following hypocaloric diets. *Ann Nutr Metab.* 2010; 57(2): 95–102.

Saavedra JM. Clinical applications of probiotic agents. *Am J Clin Nutr.* 2001; 73: 1147S–51S.

Sacks FM et al. Effects of high vs. low glycemic index of dietary carbohydrate on cardiovascular disease risk factors and insulin sensitivity. *JAMA.* 2014; 312: 2531–41.

Shahar DR et al. Does dairy calcium intake enhance weight loss among overweight diabetic patients? *Diabetes Care.* 2007; 30(3): 485–89.

Solomon CG et al. Moderate alcohol consumption and risk of coronary heart disease among women with type 2 diabetes. *Circulation.* 2000; 102: 494–99.

Taubert D et al. Effects of low habitual cocoa intake on blood pressure and bioactive nitric oxide. *JAMA.* 2007; 298: 49–60.

Thun MJ et al. Alcohol consumption and mortality among middle aged and elderly US adults. *N Engl J Med.* 1997; 337: 1705–14.

Wan Y et al. Effects of cocoa powder and dark chocolate on LDL oxidative susceptibility and prostaglandin concentrations in humans. *Am J Clin Nutr.* 2001; 74: 596–602.

Yanovski JA et al. Effects of calcium supplementation on body weight and adiposity in over-weight and obese adults: A randomized trial. *Ann Intern Med.* 2009; 150(12): 821–29, W145–46.

Zemel MB, Miller SL. Dietary calcium and dairy modulation of adiposity and obesity risk. *Nutr Rev.* 2004; 62: 125–31.

Zhang Z et al. A high legume low glycemic index diet improves serum lipid profiles in men. *Lipids.* 2010; 45: 765–75.

Chapter 8. Smart Supplements

Adams J et al. Vitamin K in the treatment and prevention of osteoporosis and arterial calcification. *Am J Health Syst Pharm.* 2005; 62: 1574–81.

Albert BB et al. Fish oil supplements in New Zealand are highly oxidized and do not meet label content of n–3 PUFA. *Sci Rep.* 2015; 5: 7928. doi: 10.1038/srep07928.

Ascherio A et al. Dietary intake of marine n–3 fatty acids, fish intake, and the risk of coronary disease among men. *N Engl J Med.* 1995; 332: 977–82.

Avogaro P et al. Acute effects of L-carnitine on FFA and beta-OH-butyrate in man. *Pharmacol Res Commun.* 1981; 13(5): 443–50.

Backes JM, Howard PA. Association of HMG-Co reductase inhibitors with neuropathy. *Ann Pharmacother.* 2003; 37: 274–78.

Basu A. Green tea supplementation affects body weight, lipids, and lipid peroxidation in obese subjects with metabolic syndrome. *J Am Coll Nutr.* 2010; 29(1): 31–40.

Bayet-Rober M et al. Phase I dose escalation trial of docetaxel plus curcumin in patients with advanced and metastatic breast cancer. *Cancer Biol Ther.* 2010; 9(1): 8–14.

Belluzzi A et al. Effect of an enteric-coated fish oil preparation on relapses in Crohn's disease. *N Engl J Med.* 1996; 334: 1557–60.

Bischoff-Ferrari HA et al. Estimation of optimal serum concentrations of 25-hydroxyvitamin D for multiple health outcomes. *Am J Clin Nutr.* 2006; 84: 18–28.

Bo S, Pisu E. Role of dietary magnesium in cardiovascular disease prevention, insulin sensitivity and diabetes. *Curr Opin Lipidol.* 2008 Feb;19(1):50–6.

Bordelon P et al. Vitamin D deficiency. *Am Fam Physician.* 2009; 80: 840–46.

Boschmann M, Thielecke F. The effects of epigallocatechin–3-gallate on thermogenesis and fat oxidation in obese men: A pilot study. *J Am Coll Nutr.* 2007; 26(4): 389S–95S.

Bowden RG et al. Fish oil supplementation lowers CRP levels independent of triglyceride reductions in patients with end stage renal disease. *Nutr Clin Pract.* 2009; 24(4): 508–12.

Chapuy MC et al. Vitamin D3 and calcium to prevent hip fractures in elderly women. *N Engl J Med.* 1992; 327: 1637–42.

Chiuve SE et al. Plasma and dietary magnesium and risk of sudden cardiac death in women. *Am J Clin Nutr.* 2011; 93: 253–60.

Cockayne S et al. Vitamin K and the prevention of fractures. *Arch Intern Med.* 2006; 166: 1256–61.

Covington MB. Omega–3 fatty acids. *Am Fam Physician.* 2004; 70(1): 133–40.

Darlington LG et al. Review of dietary therapy for rheumatoid arthritis. *Br J Rheum.* 1993; 32: 507–14.

Davis CD. Vitamin D and cancer: Current dilemmas and future research needs. *Am J Clin Nutr.* 2008; 88: 565S–69S.

De Lorgeril M et al. Mediterranean alpha-linolenic acid rich diet in secondary prevention of coronary heart disease. *Lancet.* 1994; 343: 1454–59.

Dulloo AG et al. Efficacy of a green tea extract rich in catechin polyphenols and caffeine in increasing 24-h energy expenditure and fat oxidation in humans. *Am J Clin Nutr.* 1999; 70(6): 1040–45.

Ebbing M et al. Cancer incidence and mortality after treatment with folic acid and vitamin B12. *JAMA.* 2009; 302: 2119–26.

Farzaneh-Far R et al. Association of marine omega–3 fatty acid levels with telomeric aging in patients with coronary heart disease. *JAMA.* 2010; 303: 250–57.

Freemont L. Biological effects of resveratrol. *Life Sci.* 2000; 66(8): 663–73.

Garg S et al. Evaluation of vitamin D medicines and dietary supplements and the physicochemical analysis of selected formulations. *J Nutr Health Aging.* 2013; 17: 158–61.

Garland CF et al. Can colon cancer incidence and death rates be reduced with calcium and vitamin D? *Am J Clin Nutr.* 1991; 54: 193S–203S.

———. Vitamin D for cancer prevention: Global perspective. *Ann Epidemiol.* 2009; 19: 468–83.

Gaziano JM et al. Multivitamins in the prevention of cancer in men. *JAMA.* 2012; 308: 1871–80.

Geleijnse JM et al. Inverse association of tea and flavonoid intakes with incident myocardial infarction: The Rotterdam Study. *Am J Clin Nutr.* 2002; 75: 880–86.

GISSI-Prevenzione Investigators. Vitamin E and fish oil for cardiovascular disease. *Lancet.* 1999; 354: 471.

Heaney RP. Vitamin D and calcium interactions: Functional outcomes. *Am J Clin Nutr.* 2008; 88: 541S–44S.

Heaney RP et al. Vitamin D3 distribution and status in the body. *J Am Coll Nutr.* 2009; 28: 252–56.

Heaney RP et al. Vitamin D(3) is more potent than vitamin D(2) in humans. *J Clin Endocrinol Metab.* 2011; 96(3): E447–52.

Hendler S. *PDR for Nutritional Supplements.* 2nd ed. (PDR Network, 2008), 152.

Hill AM et al. Can EGCG reduce abdominal fat in obese subjects? *J Am Coll Nutr.* 2007; 26(4): 396S–402S.

Hininger-Favier I. Green tea extract decreases oxidative stress and improves insulin sensitivity in an animal model of insulin resistance, the fructose-fed rat. *J Am Coll Nutr.* 2009 Aug;28(4): 355–61.

Hodis HN et al. Alpha-tocopherol supplementation in healthy individuals reduces low-density lipoprotein oxidation but not atherosclerosis: VEAPS. *Circulation.* 2002; 106: 1453–59.

Holick MF. The sunlight "D"ilemma: Risk of skin cancer or bone disease and muscle weakness. *Lancet.* 2001; 358: 1500–1503.

———. Vitamin D deficiency. *New Engl J Med.* 2007; 357: 266–81.

———. Vitamin D: Importance in the prevention of cancers, type 1 diabetes, heart disease, and osteoporosis. *Am J Clin Nutr.* 2004; 79: 362–71.

Holick MF, Jenkins M. *The UV Advantage* (iBooks, 2004).

Hu FB et al. Dietary intake of alpha linolenic acid and risk of fatal ischemic heart disease among women. *Am J Clin Nutr.* 1999; 69: 890–97.

———. Fish and omega–3 fatty acid intake and risk of coronary heart disease in women. *JAMA.* 2002; 287: 1815–21.

Jiao J, Effect of n–3 PUFA supplementation on cognitive function throughout the life span from infancy to old age: a systematic review and meta-analysis of randomized controlled trials. *Am J Clin Nutr.* 2014; 100(6):1422–36. doi: 10.3945/ajcn.114.095315. Epub 2014 Oct 15.

Kim YA et al. Antiproliferative effect of resveratrol in human prostate carcinoma cells. *J Med Food.* 2003; 6(4): 273–80.

Kimball SM et al. Safety of vitamin D3 in adults with multiple sclerosis. *Am J Clin Nutr.* 2007; 86: 645–51.

Kuehn BM. High calcium intake linked to heart disease, death. *JAMA*. 2013; 309(10): 972.

Lappe JM et al. Vitamin D and calcium supplementation reduces cancer risk: Results of a randomized trial. *Am J Clin Nutr*. 2007; 85: 1586–91.

Larsson SC et al. Dietary magnesium intake and risk of stroke. *Am J Clin Nutr*. 2012; 95: 362–66.

Lichtenstein AH, Russell RM. Essential nutrients: Food or supplements? *JAMA*. 2005; 294: 351–58.

Lieberman S. *Dare to Lose: 4 Simple Steps to a Better Body* (Avery/Penguin, 2002).

Liu K et al. Effect of resveratrol on glucose control and insulin sensitivity: A meta-analysis of 11 randomized controlled trials. *Am J Clin Nutr*. 2014; 99(6): 1510–19.

Lin YF et al. Curcumin inhibits tumor growth and angiogenesis in ovarian carcinoma by targeting the nuclear factor–kappa pathway. *Clin Cancer Res*. 2007; 12: 3423–30.

Logan, AC Omega–3 fatty acids and major depression: A primer for the mental health professional. Lipids Health Dis. 2004; 3: 25. Published online 2004 Nov 9. doi: 10.1186/1476–511X–3–25.

Lucock M et al. Folic acid fortification: A double-edged sword. *Curr Opin Clin Nutr Metab Care*. 2009; 12: 555–64.

Luscombe CJ et al. Exposure to ultraviolet radiation: Association with susceptibility and age at presentation with prostate cancer. *Lancet*. 2001; 358: 641–42.

Matthews RT et al. Coenzyme Q10 administration increases brain mitochondrial concentrations and exerts neuroprotective effects. *Proc Natl Acad Sci USA*. 1998; 95(15): 8802–7.

McCann JC, Ames BN. Vitamin K, an example of triage theory: Is micronutrient inadequacy linked to diseases of aging? *Am J Clin Nutr*. 2009; 90: 889–907.

Melamed ML et al. 25-Hydroxyvitamin D levels and the risk of mortality in the general population. *Arch Intern Med*. 2008; 168: 1629–37.

Merlino LA et al. Vitamin D intake is inversely associated with rheumatoid arthritis: Results from the Iowa Women's Health Study. *Arthritis Rheum*. 2004; 50(1): 72–77.

Milano F et al. Nano-curcumin inhibits proliferation of esophageal adenocarcinoma cells and enhances the T cell mediated immune response. *Front Oncol*. 2013; 3: 137.

Mischoulon D, Fava M. Docosahexanoic acid and omega–3 fatty acids in depression. *Psychiatr Clin North Am*. 2000; 23: 785–94.

Mori TA et al. Effect of omega–3 fatty acids on oxidative stress in humans. *Redox Report*. 2000; 5: 45–46.

Morris MC, Tangney CC. A potential design flaw of randomized trials of vitamin supplements. *JAMA*. 2011; 305: 1348–49.

Muhammad KI et al. Treatment with omega–3 fatty acids reduces serum C-reactive protein concentration. *Clin Lipidol*. 2011; 6: 723–29.

Narendran, R. et al. Improved Working Memory but No Effect on Striatal Vesicular Monoamine Transporter Type 2 after Omega–3 Polyunsaturated Fatty Acid Supplementation, *PLoS*, 2012: 7(10). Published online 2012 Oct 3. doi: 10.1371/journal.pone.0046832.

Paul C. "Vitamin K." Chapter 136 in Pizzorno JE, Murray MT, eds. *Textbook of Natural Medicine*. 4th ed. (Churchill Livingstone, 2012).

Pfister R et al. Plasma vitamin C predicts incident heart failure in men and women in European Prospective Investigation into Cancer and Nutrition-Norfolk prospective study. *Am Heart J*. 2011; 162(2): 246–53.

Raffield LM et al. Cross-sectional analysis of calcium intake for associations with vascular calcification and mortality in individuals with type 2 diabetes from the Diabetes Heart Study. *Am J Clin Nutr*. 2014; 100: 1029–35.

Rasmussen HS, et al. Magnesium deficiency in patients with ischemic heart disease with and without myocardial infarction uncovered by an intravenous loading test. *Arch Inter Med* 1988; 148(2): 329–32.

Rebouche CJ, Paulson DJ. Carnitine metabolism and function in humans. *Ann Rev Nutr.* 1986; 6: 41–66.

Richards JC et al. Epigallocatechin–3-gallate increases maximal oxygen uptake in adult humans. *Med Sci Sports Exerc.* 2010; 42(4): 739–44.

Rondanelli M et al. Administration of a dietary supplement (N-oleyl-phosphatidylethanolamine and epigallocatechin–3-gallate formula) enhances compliance with diet in healthy overweight subjects: A randomized controlled trial. *Br J Nutr.* 2009; 101(3): 457–64.

Rosenfeldt FL et al. Coenzyme Q10 in the treatment of hypertension: A meta-analysis of the clinical trials. *J Human Hypertens.* 2007; 21(4): 297–306.

Sahlin K. Boosting fat burning with carnitine: An old friend comes out from the shadow. *J Physiol.* 2010; 589(7): 1509–10.

Sanders TAB et al. Triglyceride-lowering effect of marine polyunsaturates in patients with hypertriglyceridemia. *Arteriosclerosis.* 1985; 5: 459–65.

Schults CV et al. Absorption, tolerability and effects on mitochondrial activity of oral coenzyme Q10 in Parkinsonian patients. *Neurology.* 1998; 50: 793–95.

———. Effects of coenzyme Q10 in early Parkinson disease. *Arch Neurol.* 2002; 59: 1541–50.

Shea MK et al. Vitamin K supplementation and progression of coronary artery calcium in older men and women. *Am J Clin Nutr.* 2009; 89: 1799–807.

Smith D et al. Is folic acid good for everyone? *Am J Clin Nutr.* 2008; 87: 517–33.

Thielecke F et al. Epigallocatechin–3-gallate and postprandial fat oxidation in overweight/obese male volunteers: A pilot study. *Eur J Clin Nutr.* 2010; 64(7): 704–13.

Tsugawa N et al. Vitamin K status of healthy Japanese women. *Am J Clin Nutr.* 2006; 83: 380–86.

Ueshima K. Magnesium and ischemic heart disease: A review of epidemiological, experimental, and clinical evidence. *Magnes Res.* 2005; 18(4): 275–84.

Ulrich CM, Potter JD. Folate and cancer: Timing is everything. *JAMA.* 2007; 297: 2408–9.

Venables MC. Green tea extract ingestion, fat oxidation, and glucose tolerance in healthy humans. *Am J Clin Nutr.* 2008; 87(3): 778–84.

Vieth R. Why the optimal requirement for vitamin D3 is probably much higher than what is officially recommended for adults. *J Steroid Biochem Mol Biol.* 2004; 89: 575–79.

Wade L et al. Alpha-tocopherol induces proantherogenic changes to HDL2 and HDL3: An in vitro and ex vivo investigation. *Atherosclerosis.* 2013; 226: 392–97.

Wainwright PE. Nutrition and behaviour: The role of n–3 fatty acids in cognitive function. *Br J Nutr.* 2000; 83: 337–39.

Wang NP et al. Curcumin promotes cardiac repair and ameliorates cardiac dysfunction following myocardial infarction. *Br J Pharmacol.* 2012; 167(7): 1550–62.

Wolfram S. Anti-obesity effects of green tea: From bedside to bench. *Mol Nutr Food Res.* 2006; 50(2): 176–87.

Xiao, Q et al. Dietary and supplemental calcium intake and cardiovascular disease mortality: the National Institutes of Health-AARP diet and health study. *JAMA Intern Med* 2013; 173(8): 639–46.

Chapter 9. Smart Living

Ayas NT et al. A prospective study of sleep duration and coronary heart disease in women. *Arch Intern Med.* 2003; 163: 205–9.

"Blue Light Has a Dark Side." Harvard Health Publications, Harvard Medical School. http://www.health.harvard.edu/staying-healthy/blue-light-has-a-dark-side.

Broussard JL et al. Impaired insulin signaling in human adipocytes after experimental sleep restriction: A randomized, crossover study. *Ann Intern Med.* 2012; 157(5): 549–57.

Buettner, D. *The Blue Zones: Lessons for Living Longer from the People Who've Lived the Longest.* National Geographic; Reprint edition (Oct 19, 2010).

Bulkeley K. Why Sleep Deprivation Is Torture. 15 Dec 2014. *Psychology Today.* https://www.psychologytoday.com/blog/dreaming-in-the-digital-age/201412/why-sleep-deprivation-is-torture.

Castillo-Richmond A et al. Effects of stress reduction on carotid atherosclerosis in hypertensive African Americans. *Stroke.* 2000; 31: 568–73.

Chaput JP. Sleeping more to improve appetite and body weight control: Dream or reality? *Am J Clin Nutr.* 2015; 101: 5–6.

Dashti HS et al. Habitual sleep duration is associated with BMI and macronutrient intake and may be modified by CLOCK genetic variants. *Am J Clin Nutr.* 2015; 101: 35–43.

Dement WC. *The Promise of Sleep* (Delacorte, 1999), 274.

Elzinga BM, Roelofs K. Cortisol-induced impairments of working memory require acute sympathetic activation. *Behav Neurosci.* 2005; 119: 98–103.

Erickson KI, Kramer AF. Aerobic exercise effects on cognitive and neural plasticity in older adults. *Br J Sports Med.* 2009; 43(1): 22–24.

Evans WJ. Effects of exercise on body composition and functional capacity of the elderly. *J Gerontol A Biol Sci Med Sci.* 1995; 50: 14–50.

Ewbank PP et al. Physical activity as a predictor of weight maintenance in previously obese subjects. *Obesity Research.* 1995; 3: 257–62.

Gallagher D et al. Healthy percentage body fat ranges: An approach for developing guidelines based on body mass index. *Am J Clin Nutr.* 2000; 72: 694–701.

Gregg EW et al. Association of an intensive lifestyle intervention with remission of type 2 diabetes. *JAMA.* 2012; 308: 2489–96.

Hambrecht R et al. Effect of exercise on coronary endothelial function in patients with coronary artery disease. *N Engl J Med.* 2000; 342: 454–60.

Irwin ML et al. Effect of exercise on total and intra-abdominal body fat in postmenopausal women. *JAMA.* 2003; 289: 323–30.

Janssen I et al. Waist circumference and not body mass index explains obesity-related health risk. *Am J Clin Nutr.* 2004; 79: 379–84.

Kramer AF et al. Ageing, fitness and neurocognitive function. *Nature.* 1999; 400(6743): 418–19.

Langer E, Rodin J. The effects of choice and enhanced personal responsibility for the aged: A field experiment in an institutional setting. *J Pers Soc Psychol.* 1976; 45(2): 191–98.

Lee IM et al. Physical activity and weight gain prevention. *JAMA.* 2010; 303: 1173–79.

Lillberg K et al. Stressful life events and risk of breast cancer in 10,808 women: A cohort study. *Am J Epidemiol.* 2003; 157(5): 415–23.

"Married People Less Likely to Have Cardiovascular Problems, According to Large-Scale Study by Researchers at NYU Langone." Newswise, NYU Langone Medical Center. 28 March 2014. http://www.newswise.com/articles/married-people-less-likely-to-have-cardiovascular-problems-according-to-large-scale-study-by-researchers-at-nyu-langone.

Myers J et al. Exercise capacity and mortality among men referred for exercise testing. *N Engl J Med.* 2002; 346: 793–80.

Parker-Pope T. "Is Marriage Good for Your Health?" *New York Times Magazine.* 14 April 2010. http://www.nytimes.com/2010/04/18/magazine/18marriage-t.html?_r=0.

Patel SR et al. Association between reduced sleep and weight gain in women. *Am J Epidemiol.* 2006; 164(10): 947–54.

Rantanen T et al. Muscle strength and body mass index as long-term predictors of mortality in initially healthy men. *J Gerontol A Biol Sci Med Sci.* 2000; 55: 168–73.

Rowe J, Kahn R. *Successful Aging* (Dell, 1998).

Schnid SM et al. A single night of sleep deprivation increases ghrelin levels and feelings of hunger in normal-weight healthy men. *J Sleep Res.* 2008; 17(3): 331–34.

Siegler IC et al. Consistency and timing of marital transitions and survival during midlife: The role of personality and health risk behaviors. *Ann Behav Med.* 2013; 45(3): 338–47.

Spiegel K et al. Effect of sleep deprivation on response to immunization. *JAMA.* 2002; 288(12): 1471–72.

Sun SS et al. Development of bioelectrical impedance analysis prediction equations for body composition with the use of a multicomponent model for use in epidemiologic surveys. *Am J Clin Nutr.* 2003; 77: 331–40.

Taheri S et al. Short sleep duration is associated with reduced leptin, elevated ghrelin, and increased body mass index. *PLoS Med.* 2004; 1(3): e62. doi: 10.1371/journal.pmed.0010062.

Traustadottir T et al. The HPA axis response to stress in women: Effects of aging and fitness. *Psychoneuroendocrinology.* 2005; 30: 392–402.

Vaillant GE. *Aging Well* (Little Brown, 2002).

Watson NF et al. A twin study of sleep duration and body mass index. *J Clin Sleep Med.* 2010; 6(1): 11–17.

Weinstein AR et al. Relationship of physical activity versus body mass index with type 2 diabetes in women. *JAMA.* 2004; 292: 1188–94.

Williams RB et al. Psychosocial risk factors for cardiovascular disease: More than one culprit at work. *JAMA.* 2003; 290: 2190–92.

Wing RR, Phelan S. Long-term weight loss maintenance. *Am J Clin Nutr.* 2005; 82(1): 2225–55.

Chapter 10: Smart Recipes

Brown LG et al. Frequency of inadequate chicken cross-contamination prevention and cooking practices in restaurants. *J Food Protection.* 2013; 76(12): 2141–45.

Acknowledgments

It is a pleasure to extend a heartfelt thank you to everyone who has helped create this book. First and foremost, I thank my wife, Nicole, for her endless support of the time and energy spent creating this book, for testing all my recipes, and for her love and devotion. A big thanks as well to my sons Lucas and Marcos for their ongoing support with creating and testing recipes and analyzing data at our clinic.

I am grateful to my very gifted new colleague and friend, Jonny Bowden. He has been an incredible writing partner and a great source of creativity in fine-tuning our unified message and empowering millions toward a Smart Fat life. I owe a special thanks to my agent, Celeste Fine, who has been inspirational and has been active throughout the book's production, including her team, especially John Maas. I feel very fortunate to have worked with Becky Cabaza, a talented writer who has provided superb guidance and artfully combined my voice with Jonny's in a clear and unified way. I owe a special thanks to the whole HarperOne team, in particular our terrific editor, Gideon Weil, who has worked to ensure our message is clear and powerful.

My mastermind group, led by JJ Virgin, has been instrumental in pushing me to create this book. I'm grateful to JJ for encouraging me to make a difference on a large scale, and thanks to the many Sapphire members, past and present, who have shared their own resources to help me create this material, including: Anna Cabeca, Alan Christianson, Leanne Ely, Sara Gottfried, and Marcelle Pick. I'm grateful as well to Ellyne Lonergan for fine-tuning my message with PBS, which has impacted this book in many ways.

My current medical team at the Masley Optimal Health Center has been incredible in their support for this manuscript, with special thanks to Nicole Masley, Angie Presby, Katherine Reay, and James Porcelli, plus extra thanks to my office coordinator, Kim Escarraz, who has played an invaluable role in supporting everything I do. Thanks to several physician colleagues who helped my research for this book, namely Douglas Schocken and Richard Roetzheim, and my medical library team at Morton Plant Hospital: Karen Roth and Rachelle Benzarti. Plus, thanks to my Functional Medicine mentors who have provided the backbone of my clinical education, including Jeffrey Bland, Mark Hyman, and David Perlmutter.

Many thanks to my recipe testers for helping me make them delicious and easy to follow—Gordon Wheat, Megan Hubbard, Julia Sokoloff, Michelle and Gary Crosby, plus my family testers—Brooke Masley, Evelyn Odegaard, Peggy and Arp Masley, and Susan Thomas.

—*Steven Masley*

My favorite part of writing a book is when I get to write the acknowledgments, because it's a rare opportunity to tell all the people in your life how you feel about them and how much you appreciate them.

I am beyond blessed to have had the opportunity to work with Dr. Steven Masley, a textbook example of a true healer: brilliant, caring, and dedicated. And to have had nearly fifteen years of being represented by the most wonderful and dedicated agent anyone could ask for—Coleen O'Shea of Allen O'Shea. And to have an editor as passionate, supportive, and skillful as Gideon Weil.

Over the years, I've been fortunate to work with wonderful companies—especially Barleans (and Bruce Barlean particularly), Reserveage (Naomi Whittel), Europharma (Terry Lemerond, Cheryl Meyers, Kathy

Arendt), VRP (Kelly Cleary, Kevin O'Donohue, Kimberly Day), Natural Health Sherpa (Marc Stockman, Jeff Radich, Dr. Dean Raffelock).

JJ Virgin—whose vision created the greatest mastermind group on the planet, the Mindshare Summit—and a special thanks to all the members of the Sapphire Group, past and present, for all your support and inspiration.

My brilliant and visionary social media strategist (and friend) Mary Agnes Antonpoulos, her partner Tommy, and their company, Viral Integrity.

Mike Danielson and his team at Media Relations: Heather Stetler, Heather Arre, Heather Champine, Gail Brandt, Krista Wignall, Robin Miller.

The three writers who have influenced me the most: Ed McBain, William Goldman, Robert Sapolsky.

Dean Draznin and his team at Dean Draznin Communications (thanks, Diane!).

Becky Cabaza—This book might have been written without Becky, but it would have been nowhere near as good. Thank you for your patient and wise counsel, and your enormous talents—as a writer and editor and part-time therapist.

My absolutely indefatigable assistant (and friend), who makes my life work: Amber Linder. And to the others who help her in the thankless job of keeping me on track and organized, a task that's been said to have a disturbing similarity to herding a pack of Jack Russell terriers: Brooke Baird, Gabriella Periera, Chad Ellington, Jeannette Boudreau, Robert Kernochan, Scott Nelson, and Pamela Kostas. I appreciate all of you so very much.

My Los Angeles family: Sky London, Doug Monas, Bootsie, Zack, Sage and Luke Grakal. I love you all.

And to the following people, each of whom has given me a gift for which I am deeply and eternally grateful: Oliver Becault, Jeannette Bessinger, Cadence Bowden, Jeffrey Bowden, Pace Bowden, Peter Breger, Anja Christy, Drew Christy, Christopher Crabb, Lauree Dash, Glen and Dawn Depke, Christopher Duncan, Taryn Sena Dunivant, Scott Ellis, Oz Garcia, Nancy Feidler, Jared Gilmore, Randy Graff, Pam Hendrikson, Jade Hochanadel, Zoe Hochanadel, Kevin Hogan, Harlan and Sandy Kleiman, Mike Koenigs, Dr. Dave Leonardi, Dr. Richard Lewis, Amber Linder, Sky London, Liz Neporent, Marianna Riccio, Ed Rush, Billy Stritch, Dr. Beth Traylor, Danny Troob, Lauren Trotter, Al Waxman, Anita Waxman, Susan Wood, Ketura Worthen.

And, of course, to Michelle—the great love of my life, forever my *beschert*. I love you.

—Jonny Bowden

Recipe Index

almond butter: Chicken Satay Skewers
with Cabbage Wraps, 255–56;
Chocolate, Cherry, and Spinach
Shake, 232; Smart Fat Shake, 229

almond milk: Chocolate and Strawberry
Shake, 232; Chocolate, Cherry, and
Spinach Shake, 232; Smart Fat Shake,
229; Smart Fat Steel-Cut Oatmeal,
235; Vanilla, Blueberry, and Spinach
Shake, 231

almond oil: Broiled Oysters with
Walnut, Parmesan Cheese, and
Parsley Crust, 269; Fruit and Nut
Crumble, 284; Sautéed Kale with
Garlic and Lemon, 278; Steak
Kebobs with Pineapple, Onion,
and Bell Pepper, 261–62; Wild Rice
and Quinoa with Kale and Slivered
Almonds, 280–81

almonds: Avocado, Cucumber, and
Garbanzo Salad, 240; Baked Halibut
with Almond Crust, 271; Cherry-
Ricotta Swirl, 281; Fruit and Nut
Crumble, 281; Moroccan Chicken
Stew, 249–50; Mushroom-Nut Pâté,
272; Smart Fat Steel-Cut Oatmeal,
235; Wild Mushroom Soufflé, 275–76;
Wild Rice and Quinoa with Kale and
Slivered Almonds, 280–81

appetizers. See snacks and appetizers

apples: Dark Chocolate Drizzle, 282–83;
Fruit and Nut Crumble, 284

artichoke hearts: Frittata, 234;
Marinated Flank Steak over Mixed

Green Salad, 259–60

Arugula, Shrimp, Fennel, and
Cannellini Bean Salad with Orange
Vinaigrette, 241–42

Asian Pear, Gorgonzola Cheese,
Walnuts, and Raspberries, 237

Avocado, Cucumber, and Garbanzo
Salad, 240

avocados: Avocado, Cucumber, and
Garbanzo Salad, 240; Ceviche,
267–68; Crab Avocado Dip, 237–38;
Cucumber with Smoked Oysters
and Avocado, 236; Guacamole with
Jicama and Red Bell Pepper, 239;
hastening the ripening process of,
226; Lump Crab and Mango-Avocado
Salsa, 238; as smart fat staple, 226

Baked Halibut with Almond Crust, 271

Baked White Fish with Orange
Marinade, 264–65

basil: keep fresh supply on hand, 222;
Roasted Grass-Fed Bison and Root
Vegetables, 257–58

beans: keep supply of, 241–42; Sirloin
Steak Chili, 258–59; Soup of the
Week, 245–46; Turkey Meatballs,
250–51; Wild Rice and Quinoa with
Kale and Slivered Almonds, 280–81

beef. See meat/meat dishes

Beef Stew, 262–63

beets: Borscht, 244–45; Roasted Grass-
Fed Bison and Root Vegetables,
257–58

bell peppers: Ceviche, 267–68; Steak Kebobs with Pineapple, Onion, and Bell Pepper, 261–62

berries: Asian Pear, Gorgonzola Cheese, Walnuts, and Raspberries, 237; Smart Fat Shake, 229; Smart Fat Steel-Cut Oatmeal, 235

blackberries (Fruit and Nut Crumble), 284

blueberries, Vanilla, Blueberry, and Spinach Shake, 231

Borscht, 244–45

breakfast dishes: Chocolate and Strawberry Shake, 232; Chocolate, Cherry, and Spinach Shake, 232; Frittata, 234; Omelet with Sweet Onion, Red Bell Pepper, and Kale, 233; Smart Fat Shakes (basic) and variation tips, 229–30; Smart Fat Steel-Cut Oatmeal, 235; Vanilla, Blueberry, and Spinach Shake, 231; Vanilla, Cherry, and Kale Shake, 231

broccoli, Coconut Milk Curry with Shrimp and Broccoli, 266–67

Broiled Oysters with Walnut, Parmesan Cheese, and Parsley Crust, 269

broths: Beef Stew, 262–63; Borscht, 244–45; Butternut Squash Soup with Ginger and Fennel, 246–47; to keep in your pantry, 225; Lentil Curry, 273; Soup of the Week, 245–46; Wild Rice and Quinoa with Kale and Slivered Almonds, 280–81. *See also* stocks

Brussels Sprouts with Smart Lemon-Butter Sauce, 278–79

butter: Baked White Fish with Orange Marinade, 264–65; Baked Halibut with Almond Crust, 271; Brussels Sprouts with Smart Lemon-Butter Sauce, 278–79; clarified, 262–63; Crab Cakes with Quinoa, 265–66; Dark Chocolate Drizzle, 282–83; Fruit and Nut Crumble, 284; Salmon with Smart Lemon-Butter Sauce, 270. *See also* nut butters

Butternut Squash Soup with Ginger and Fennel, 246–47

cabbage: Borscht, 244–45; Chicken Satay Skewers with Cabbage Wraps, 255–56; Moroccan Chicken Stew, 249–50; Steak Kebobs with Pineapple, Onion, and Bell Pepper, 261–62

canned or jarred staples, 225

cannellini beans (Shrimp, Fennel, and Cannellini Bean Salad with Orange Vinaigrette), 241–42

caraway seeds (Borscht), 244–45

cardamom: keep supply of, 221; Middle Eastern Chicken Sauté, 254

carrots: Beef Stew, 262–63; Borscht, 244–45; Crab Cakes with Quinoa, 265–66

Sirloin Steak Chili, 258–59; Soup of the Week, 245–46; White Bean Salad, 242–43

cauliflower (Vegetable Korma), 274

cayenne pepper supply, 221

celery: Beef Stew, 262–63; Borscht, 244–45; Crab Cakes with Quinoa, 265–66; Lentil Curry, 273; Moroccan Chicken Stew, 249–50; Sirloin Steak Chili, 258–59; Soup of the Week, 245–46; White Bean Salad, 242–43

Ceviche, 267–68

cheese: Asian Pear, Gorgonzola Cheese, Walnuts, and Raspberries, 237; Broiled Oysters with Walnut, Parmesan Cheese, and Parsley Crust, 269; Frittata, 234; Mushroom-Nut Pâté, 272; Omelet with Sweet Onion, Red Bell Pepper, and Kale, 233; Parmesan (or Parmigiano-Reggiano) cheese, 225, 233; Shrimp, Fennel, and Cannellini Bean Salad with Orange Vinaigrette, 241–42; Turkey Meatballs, 250–51; White Bean Salad, 242–43; Wild Mushroom Soufflé, 275–76; Wild Rice and Quinoa with Kale and Slivered Almonds, 280–81

cherries: Cherry-Ricotta Swirl, 281; Chocolate, Cherry, and Spinach Shake, 232; Dark Chocolate Drizzle, 282–83; Vanilla, Cherry, and Kale Shake, 231; Cherry-Ricotta Swirl, 281

chia seeds: Smart Fat Shake, 229;
Vanilla, Cherry, and Kale Shake, 231
Chicken Satay Skewers with Cabbage
Wraps, 255–56
Chicken with Pecan-Herb Crust, 252
chives (Borscht), 244–45
Chocolate and Strawberry Shake, 232
Chocolate, Cherry, and Spinach
Shake, 232
cilantro: Ceviche, 267–68; Coconut Milk
Curry with Shrimp and Broccoli,
266–67; Cucumber with Smoked
Oysters and Avocado, 236; Guacamole
with Jicama and Red Bell Pepper, 239;
keep fresh supply on hand, 222; Lump
Crab and Mango-Avocado Salsa, 238;
Raita, 275; Sirloin Steak Chili, 258–59;
Tandoori Chicken, 253–54; Vegetable
Korma, 274
cinnamon: Fruit and Nut Crumble, 284;
keep supply of, 221; Middle Eastern
Chicken Sauté, 254; Moroccan
Chicken Stew, 249–50; Pumpkin
Pudding, 282; Smart Fat Steel-Cut
Oatmeal, 235
clarified butter: Beef Stew, 262–63;
cooking technique for, 263; Clean
Fifteen produce list, 226
coconut milk: Chicken Satay Skewers
with Cabbage Wraps, 255–56;
Coconut Milk Curry with Shrimp
and Broccoli, 266–67; Lentil Curry,
273; Moroccan Chicken Stew, 249–50;
pantry supply of, 225
Coconut Milk Curry with Shrimp and
Broccoli, 266–67
coconut oil: Chicken Satay Skewers
with Cabbage Wraps, 255–56;
Coconut Milk Curry with Shrimp and
Broccoli, 266–67; Lentil Curry, 273
cooking techniques: clarifying butter,
263; food safety, 227; oil cooking temperatures and smoke point, 223–24
Crab Avocado Dip, 237–38
Crab Cakes with Quinoa, 265–66
crab dishes: Crab Avocado Dip, 237–38;
Lump Crab and Mango-Avocado
Salsa, 238

cream: Butternut Squash Soup with
Ginger and Fennel, 246–47; Fruit
and Nut Crumble, 281; Pumpkin
Pudding, 282
crushed red pepper flakes: keep supply
of, 221; Sirloin Steak Chili, 258–59
cucumbers: Avocado, Cucumber,
and Garbanzo Salad, 240; Ceviche,
267–68; Cucumber with Smoked
Oysters and Avocado, 236; Lump
Crab and Mango-Avocado Salsa,
238; Raita, 275
Cucumber with Smoked Oysters and
Avocado, 236
curry spice blend: Butternut Squash
Soup with Ginger and Fennel, 246–47;
Coconut Milk Curry with Shrimp and
Broccoli, 266–67; keep pantry supply
of, 221; Lentil Curry, 273; Moroccan
Chicken Stew, 249–50; Tandoori
Chicken, 253–54; Vegetable
Korma, 274

dairy supplies, 225. *See also specific
dairy product*
dark chocolate: Dark Chocolate Drizzle,
282–83; pantry supply of, 225
Dark Chocolate Drizzle, 282–83
Desserts: Cherry-Ricotta Swirl, 281;
Dark Chocolate Drizzle, 282–83;
Fruit and Nut Crumble, 284; Fruit
Salad with Mint, Lemon Rind,
and Greek Yogurt, 283; Pumpkin
Pudding, 282
dill weed: Borscht, 244–45; keep supply
of, 221
Dirty Dozen produce list, 226

eggs: Baked Halibut with Almond Crust,
271; Broiled Oysters with Walnut,
Parmesan Cheese, and Parsley
Crust, 269; Chicken with Pecan-Herb
Crust, 252; Crab Cakes with Quinoa,
265–66; Frittata, 234; Mushroom-
Nut Pâté, 272; Omelet with Sweet
Onion, Red Bell Pepper, and Kale,
233; Pumpkin Pudding, 282; Turkey
Meatballs, 250–51

Environmental Working Group's Dirty Dozen and Clean Fifteen lists, 226

extra-virgin olive oil: Brussels Sprouts with Smart Lemon-Butter Sauce, 278–79; Ceviche, 267–68; Marinated Flank Steak over Mixed Green Salad, 259–60; Purple Potatoes with Garlic, Herbs, and Parsley, 277; Salmon with Smart Lemon-Butter Sauce, 270; Smart Vinaigrette Dressing, 243; Steak Kebobs with Pineapple, Onion, and Bell Pepper, 261–62; when to and when not to use, 222. *See also* olive oil

fennel: Butternut Squash Soup with Ginger and Fennel, 246–47; Shrimp, Fennel, and Cannellini Bean Salad with Orange Vinaigrette, 241–42

fines herbes: keep supply of, 221; Roasted Grass-Fed Bison and Root Vegetables, 257–58; Wild Mushroom Soufflé, 275–76

flavors: fresh flavors to have on hand, 221–22; oils for salad dressings and drizzling for additional, 223–24; "smart spice rack" list, 221

food safety tips: buying fresh seafood, 264; on storing and cooking meat, poultry, fish, 226–27

freezer items: frozen fruits and veggies, 227; poultry, meat, fish, 227–28. *See also* pantry items

Frittata, 234

frozen fruits and veggies, 227

fruit: Dark Chocolate Drizzle, 282–83; frozen, 227; Fruit and Nut Crumble, 284; Fruit Salad with Mint, Lemon Rind, and Greek Yogurt, 283; keeping pantry supply of, 225; organic vs. not organic debate, 226; Smart Fat Steel-Cut Oatmeal, 235. *See also specific fruit*

Fruit and Nut Crumble, 284

Fruit Salad with Mint, Lemon Rind, and Greek Yogurt, 283

garbanzo beans: Soup of the Week, 245–46; Turkey Meatballs, 250–51;

Wild Rice and Quinoa with Kale and Slivered Almonds, 280–81

garlic cloves: Avocado, Cucumber, and Garbanzo Salad, 240; Borscht, 244–45; Brussels Sprouts with Smart Lemon-Butter Sauce, 278–79; Chicken Satay Skewers with Cabbage Wraps, 255–56; Chicken with Pecan-Herb Crust, 252; Coconut Milk Curry with Shrimp and Broccoli, 266–67; Cucumber with Smoked Oysters and Avocado, 236; keep fresh supply on hand, 221; Lentil Curry, 273; Marinated Flank Steak over Mixed Green Salad, 259–60; Middle Eastern Chicken Sauté, 254; Purple Potatoes with Garlic, Herbs, and Parsley, 277; Roasted Grass-Fed Bison and Root Vegetables, 257–58; Salmon with Smart Lemon-Butter Sauce, 270; Sautéed Kale with Garlic and Lemon, 278; Sautéed Swiss Chard with Garlic and Italian Herbs, 279; Shrimp, Fennel, and Cannellini Bean Salad with Orange Vinaigrette, 241–42; Smart Vinaigrette Dressing, 243; Steak Kebobs with Pineapple, Onion, and Bell Pepper, 261–62; Vegetable Korma, 274; White Bean Salad, 242–43

gingerroot: Butternut Squash Soup with Ginger and Fennel, 246–47; Chicken Satay Skewers with Cabbage Wraps, 255–56; Coconut Milk Curry with Shrimp and Broccoli, 266–67; keep fresh supply on hand, 221; Lentil Curry, 273; Middle Eastern Chicken Sauté, 254; Pumpkin Pudding, 282; Tandoori Chicken, 253–54; Vegetable Korma, 274

gluten-free tamari supply, 225

grains: Coconut Milk Curry with Shrimp and Broccoli, 266–67; Crab Cakes with Quinoa, 265–66; pantry supply of, 225; Wild Rice and Quinoa with Kale and Slivered Almonds, 280–81

green onions: Ceviche, 267–68; Frittata,

234; Lump Crab and Mango-Avocado Salsa, 238; Turkey Meatballs, 250–51
Grilled Lamb Chops, 260–61
Gruyère cheese: Frittata, 234; Mushroom-Nut Pâté, 272; Wild Mushroom Soufflé, 275–76
Guacamole with Jicama and Red Bell Pepper, 239

herbs and spices: fresh flavors to have on hand, 221–22; "smart spice rack" list of, 221. *See also specific herb and spice*
heterocyclic amines: as cancer-causing compounds, 227
hot chili sauce: Broiled Oysters with Walnut, Parmesan Cheese, and Parsley Crust, 269; Chicken Satay Skewers with Cabbage Wraps, 255–56; pantry supply of, 225; Steak Kebobs with Pineapple, Onion, and Bell Pepper, 261–62

Italian herbs: Chicken with Pecan-Herb Crust, 252; how to shop for, 221; Marinated Flank Steak over Mixed Green Salad, 259–60; Purple Potatoes with Garlic, Herbs, and Parsley, 277; Roasted Chicken with Mediterranean Herbs, 248; Roasted Grass-Fed Bison and Root Vegetables, 257–58; Sautéed Swiss Chard with Garlic and Italian Herbs, 279; Sautéed Turkey Loins with Italian Herbs, 251; Soup of the Week, 245–46; Turkey Meatballs, 250–51; White Bean Salad, 242; Wild Rice and Quinoa with Kale and Slivered Almonds, 280–81
Italian parsley: Avocado, Cucumber, and Garbanzo Salad, 240; Baked White Fish with Orange Marinade, 264–65; Broiled Oysters with Walnut, Parmesan Cheese, and Parsley Crust, 269; Coconut Milk Curry with Shrimp and Broccoli, 266–67; Crab Avocado Dip, 237–38; Cucumber with Smoked Oysters and Avocado, 236; Omelet with Sweet Onion, Red Bell Pepper,

and Kale, 233; Purple Potatoes with Garlic, Herbs, and Parsley, 277; Roasted Grass-Fed Bison and Root Vegetables, 257–58; Tandoori Chicken, 253–54; Turkey Meatballs, 250–51; White Bean Salad, 242–43; Wild Mushroom Soufflé, 275–76. *See also* parsley

jicama root: Ceviche, 267–68; Guacamole with Jicama and Red Bell Pepper, 239

kale leaves: Omelet with Sweet Onion, Red Bell Pepper, and Kale, 233; Sautéed Kale with Garlic and Lemon, 278; Smart Fat Shake, 229; Vanilla, Cherry, and Kale Shake, 231
kitchen essentials list, 228

lamb. *See* meats/meat dishes
lemons: Brussels Sprouts with Smart Lemon-Butter Sauce, 278–79; Cherry-Ricotta Swirl, 281; Crab Cakes with Quinoa, 265–66; Fruit Salad with Mint, Lemon Rind, and Greek Yogurt, 283; Salmon with Smart Lemon-Butter Sauce, 270; Sautéed Kale with Garlic and Lemon, 278; Tandoori Chicken, 253–54
Lentil Curry, 273
Lump Crab and Mango-Avocado Salsa, 238

main dishes: Baked Halibut with Almond Crust, 271; Baked White Fish with Orange Marinade, 264–65; Beef Stew, 262–63; Broiled Oysters with Walnut, Parmesan Cheese, and Parsley Crust, 269; Ceviche, 267–68; Chicken Satay Skewers with Cabbage Wraps, 255–56; Chicken with Pecan-Herb Crust, 252; Coconut Milk Curry with Shrimp and Broccoli, 266–67; Crab Cakes with Quinoa, 265–66; Grilled Lamb Chops, 260–61; Lentil Curry, 273; Marinated Flank Steak over Mixed Green Salad, 259–60;

main dishes *(continued)*
Middle Eastern Chicken Sauté, 254;
Moroccan Chicken Stew, 249–50;
Mushroom-Nut Pâté, 272; Raita, 275;
Roasted Chicken with Mediterranean
Herbs, 248; Roasted Grass-Fed
Bison and Root Vegetables, 257–58;
Salmon with Smart Lemon-Butter
Sauce, 270; Sautéed Turkey Loins
with Italian Herbs, 251; Sirloin Steak
Chili, 258–59; Steak Kebobs with
Pineapple, Onion, and Bell Pepper,
261–62; Tandoori Chicken, 253–54;
Turkey Meatballs, 250–51; Vegetable
Korma, 274; Wild Mushroom Soufflé,
275–76
mangos (Lump Crab and Mango-
Avocado Salsa), 238
maple syrup: Cherry-Ricotta Swirl, 281;
Fruit and Nut Crumble, 284
marinara sauce (Turkey Meatballs),
250–51
Marinated Flank Steak over Mixed
Green Salad, 259–60
marinating: Marinated Flank Steak over
Mixed Green Salad, 259–60; reducing
heterocyclic amines by, 227
MCT oil: Chocolate and Strawberry
Shake, 232; Smart Fat Shake, 229
meats/meat dishes: Beef Stew, 262–63;
Borscht, 244–45; food safety note on,
226–27; Grilled Lamb Chops, 260–61;
keeping a supply of, 226; Marinated
Flank Steak over Mixed Green Salad,
259–60; note on cooking techniques
for, 227; Roasted Grass-Fed Bison and
Root Vegetables, 257–58; Sirloin Steak
Chili, 258–59; Steak Kebobs with
Pineapple, Onion, and Bell Pepper,
261–62; stocking the freezer with, 227
Middle Eastern Chicken Sauté, 254
milk: Butternut Squash Soup with
Ginger and Fennel, 246–47; Frittata,
234; keeping pantry supply of, 225;
Moroccan Chicken Stew, 249–50;
Pumpkin Pudding, 282; Smart Fat
Steel-Cut Oatmeal, 235
mint: Fruit Salad with Mint, Lemon

Rind, and Greek Yogurt, 283; Grilled
Lamb Chops, 260–61; keep fresh
supply on hand, 222; Moroccan
Chicken Stew, 249–50
Moroccan Chicken Stew, 249–50
Mushroom-Nut Pâté, 272
mushrooms: Frittata, 234; Mushroom-
Nut Pâté, 272; Soup of the Week,
245–46; Wild Mushroom Soufflé,
275–76
must-have kitchen essentials list, 228

nut butters: almond butter, 229, 232,
255, 255–56; pantry supply of, 225.
See also butter
nut oil: Butternut Squash Soup with
Ginger and Fennel, 246–47; Chicken
with Pecan-Herb Crust, 252
nuts: Asian Pear, Gorgonzola Cheese,
Walnuts, and Raspberries, 237;
Dark Chocolate Drizzle, 282–83;
Mushroom-Nut Pâté, 272; pantry
supply of, 225; Smart Fat Steel-Cut
Oatmeal, 235. *See also specific type
of nut*

oil cooking temperatures: high heat,
223, 224; low heat, 223, 224; medium
heat, 223, 224; medium to high heat,
223, 224; smoke point of, 223, 224
oils: appropriate for specific cooking
temperature, 223; extra-virgin olive
oil, 222; salad dressings and drizzling
for additional flavor, 223–24;
tips for choosing the right, 222;
understanding the smoke point of,
223, 224. *See also specific type of oil*
okra (Vegetable Korma), 274
olive oil: cooking with, 222; Crab Cakes
with Quinoa, 265–66; Grilled Lamb
Chops, 260–61; Marinated Flank
Steak over Mixed Green Salad, 259–
60; Middle Eastern Chicken Sauté,
254; Moroccan Chicken Stew, 249–50;
Roasted Chicken with Mediterranean
Herbs, 248; Roasted Grass-Fed Bison
and Root Vegetables, 257–58; Sautéed
Swiss Chard with Garlic and Italian

Herbs, 279; Sautéed Turkey Loins with Italian Herbs, 251; Sirloin Steak Chili, 258–59; Soup of the Week, 245–46; Turkey Meatballs, 250–51; Wild Mushroom Soufflé, 275–76. *See also* extra-virgin olive oil

Omelet with Sweet Onion, Red Bell Pepper, and Kale, 233

onions: Beef Stew, 262–63; Butternut Squash Soup with Ginger and Fennel, 246–47; Chicken Satay Skewers with Cabbage Wraps, 255–56; Crab Cakes with Quinoa, 265–66; Guacamole with Jicama and Red Bell Pepper, 239; Lentil Curry, 273; Middle Eastern Chicken Sauté, 254; Moroccan Chicken Stew, 249–50; Mushroom-Nut Pâté, 272; Omelet with Sweet Onion, Red Bell Pepper, and Kale, 233; Raita, 275; Roasted Grass-Fed Bison and Root Vegetables, 257–58; Sirloin Steak Chili, 258–59; Soup of the Week, 245–46; Steak Kebobs with Pineapple, Onion, and Bell Pepper, 261–62; Tandoori Chicken, 253–54; Turkey Meatballs, 250–51; Vegetable Korma, 274; White Bean Salad, 242–43; Wild Rice and Quinoa with Kale and Slivered Almonds, 280–81. *See also* green onions

oranges: Baked White Fish with Orange Marinade, 264–65; Dark Chocolate Drizzle, 282–83; Fruit and Nut Crumble, 284; Shrimp, Fennel, and Cannellini Bean Salad with Orange Vinaigrette, 241–42

oregano: keep supply of, 221; Sirloin Steak Chili, 258–59

organic vs. not organic produce debate, 226

oysters: Broiled Oysters with Walnut, Parmesan Cheese, and Parsley Crust, 269; Cucumber with Smoked Oysters and Avocado, 236

pantry items: broths, 225; canned or jarred staples, 225; coconut milk, 225; dairy items, 225; dark chocolate, 225; grains, 225; herbs and spices, 221–22; nuts and nut butters, 225; poultry, meat, fish, 226–27; produce, 225–26; protein powder, 225; the right oils, 222–24; vinegars and sauces, 225. *See also* freezer items; *specific pantry item*

paprika: Baked White Fish with Orange Marinade, 264–65; Chicken Satay Skewers with Cabbage Wraps, 255–56; Coconut Milk Curry with Shrimp and Broccoli, 266–67; Crab Cakes with Quinoa, 265–66; keep supply of ground, 221; Lentil Curry, 273; Sautéed Swiss Chard with Garlic and Italian Herbs, 279; Sautéed Turkey Loins with Italian Herbs, 251; Sirloin Steak Chili, 258–59; Steak Kebobs with Pineapple, Onion, and Bell Pepper, 261–62; Tandoori Chicken, 253–54; Wild Rice and Quinoa with Kale and Slivered Almonds, 280–81

Parmesan (or Parmigiano-Reggiano) cheese: Broiled Oysters with Walnut, Parmesan Cheese, and Parsley Crust, 269; keeping pantry supply of, 225; Mushroom-Nut Pâté, 272; Omelet with Sweet Onion, Red Bell Pepper, and Kale, 233; Shrimp, Fennel, and Cannellini Bean Salad with Orange Vinaigrette, 241–42; Turkey Meatballs, 250–51; White Bean Salad, 242–43; Wild Mushroom Soufflé, 275–76; Wild Rice and Quinoa with Kale and Slivered Almonds, 280–81

parsley: keep fresh supply on hand, 222; Sautéed Swiss Chard with Garlic and Italian Herbs, 279; Sautéed Turkey Loins with Italian Herbs, 251. *See also* Italian parsley

pears: Asian Pear, Gorgonzola Cheese, Walnuts, and Raspberries, 237; Fruit and Nut Crumble, 284

peas: Chicken Satay Skewers with Cabbage Wraps, 255–56; Vegetable Korma, 274

pecan oil: Chicken with Pecan-Herb

pecan oil *(continued)*
    Crust, 252; Mushroom-Nut Pâté, 272;
    Vegetable Korma, 274; Wild Rice
    and Quinoa with Kale and Slivered
    Almonds, 280–81
pecans: Chicken with Pecan-Herb
    Crust, 252; Fruit and Nut Crumble,
    281; Mushroom-Nut Pâté, 272
pepper: ground cayenne pepper, 221;
    whole black peppercorns, 221
pineapples (Steak Kebobs with
    Pineapple, Onion, and Bell Pepper),
    261–62
pinto beans (Sirloin Steak Chili), 258–59
pistachio nuts: Fruit Salad with Mint,
    Lemon Rind, and Greek Yogurt, 283;
    Vegetable Korma, 274
potatoes: Borscht, 244–45; Purple
    Potatoes with Garlic, Herbs, and
    Parsley, 277; Soup of the Week,
    245–46
poultry: Chicken Satay Skewers with
    Cabbage Wraps, 255–56; Chicken
    with Pecan-Herb Crust, 252; food
    safety note on, 226–27; keeping
    a supply of, 226; Middle Eastern
    Chicken Sauté, 254; Moroccan
    Chicken Stew, 249–50; note on
    cooking techniques for, 227; Roasted
    Chicken with Mediterranean Herbs,
    248; Sautéed Turkey Loins with
    Italian Herbs, 251; stocking the
    freezer with, 227; Tandoori Chicken,
    253–54; Turkey Meatballs, 250–51
produce: Dirty Dozen and Clean
    Fifteen lists on, 226; frozen fruits
    and veggies, 227; organic vs. not
    organic debate on, 226; pantry supply
    of, 225–26. *See also specific fruit or
    vegetable*
protein powder: pantry supply of,
    225; Smart Fat Shakes: basic and
    variations, 229–32; Smart Fat Steel-
    Cut Oatmeal, 235
Pumpkin Pudding, 282
purple potatoes: Borscht, 244–45;
    Purple Potatoes with Garlic, Herbs,
    and Parsley, 277

Purple Potatoes with Garlic, Herbs, and
    Parsley, 277

quinoa: Crab Cakes with Quinoa,
    265–66; Wild Rice and Quinoa with
    Kale and Slivered Almonds, 280–81

Raita, 275
raspberries: Asian Pear, Gorgonzola
    Cheese, Walnuts, and Raspberries,
    237; Fruit and Nut Crumble, 281, 284
red bell peppers: Ceviche, 267–68;
    Chicken Satay Skewers with Cabbage
    Wraps, 255–56; Guacamole with
    Jicama and Red Bell Pepper, 239;
    Lump Crab and Mango-Avocado
    Salsa, 238; Omelet with Sweet Onion,
    Red Bell Pepper, and Kale, 233; Steak
    Kebobs with Pineapple, Onion,
    and Bell Pepper, 261–62; Vegetable
    Korma, 274
red cabbage (Borscht), 244–45
red pepper flakes, 221
rice: Coconut Milk Curry with Shrimp
    and Broccoli, 266–67; Wild Rice
    and Quinoa with Kale and Slivered
    Almonds, 280–81
ricotta cheese (Cherry-Ricotta Swirl), 281
Roasted Chicken with Mediterranean
    Herbs, 248
Roasted Grass-Fed Bison and Root
    Vegetables, 257–58
rolled oat (Fruit and Nut Crumble), 281
rosemary: Beef Stew, 262–63; Grilled
    Lamb Chops, 260–61; keep fresh
    supply on hand, 222

salads: Avocado, Cucumber, and
    Garbanzo Salad, 240; Shrimp, Fennel,
    and Cannellini Bean Salad with
    Orange Vinaigrette, 241–42; Smart
    Vinaigrette Dressing, 243; White
    Bean Salad, 242–43
Salmon with Smart Lemon-Butter
    Sauce, 270
sauces: gluten-free tamari, 225, 255–56,
    259–60, 260; hot chili sauce, 225,
    255–56, 261–62, 269; marinara,

250–51; Smart Lemon-Butter Sauce, 278–79

Sautéed Kale with Garlic and Lemon, 278

Sautéed Swiss Chard with Garlic and Italian Herbs, 279

Sautéed Turkey Loins with Italian Herbs, 251

seafood/seafood dishes: Baked Halibut with Almond Crust, 271; Baked White Fish with Orange Marinade, 264–65; Broiled Oysters with Walnut, Parmesan Cheese, and Parsley Crust, 269; buying fresh seafood, 264; Ceviche, 267–68; Coconut Milk Curry with Shrimp and Broccoli, 266–67; Crab Avocado Dip, 237–38; Crab Cakes with Quinoa, 265–66; Cucumber with Smoked Oysters and Avocado, 236; food safety note on fish and, 226–27; keeping a supply of fish, 226; Lump Crab and Mango-Avocado Salsa, 238; note on cooking techniques for fish, 227; Salmon with Smart Lemon-Butter Sauce, 270; Shrimp, Fennel, and Cannellini Bean Salad with Orange Vinaigrette, 241–42; stocking the freezer with vacuum-packed fish, 228

sea salt supply, 221

shallots: Grilled Lamb Chops, 260–61; Wild Mushroom Soufflé, 275–76

shrimp dishes: Coconut Milk Curry with Shrimp and Broccoli, 266–67; Shrimp, Fennel, and Cannellini Bean Salad with Orange Vinaigrette, 241–42

side dishes: Brussels Sprouts with Smart Lemon-Butter Sauce, 278–79; Purple Potatoes with Garlic, Herbs, and Parsley, 277; Sautéed Kale with Garlic and Lemon, 278; Sautéed Swiss Chard with Garlic and Italian Herbs, 279; Wild Rice and Quinoa with Kale and Slivered Almonds, 280–81

Sirloin Steak Chili, 258–59

Smart Fat Shakes: basic recipe for, 229; Chocolate and Strawberry Shake, 232; Chocolate, Cherry, and Spinach Shake, 232; tips for making variations of the basic, 230; Vanilla, Blueberry, and Spinach Shake, 231; Vanilla, Cherry, and Kale Shake, 231

Smart Fat Steel-Cut Oatmeal, 235

Smart Lemon-Butter Sauce, 278–79

Smart Vinaigrette Dressing, 243

smoke point: guide on maximum oil cooking temperatures and, 224; understanding oil, 223, 224

snacks and appetizers: Asian Pear, Gorgonzola Cheese, Walnuts, and Raspberries, 237; Crab Avocado Dip, 237–38; Cucumber with Smoked Oysters and Avocado, 236; Guacamole with Jicama and Red Bell Pepper, 239; Lump Crab and Mango-Avocado Salsa, 238

snow peas (Chicken Satay Skewers with Cabbage Wraps), 255–56

Soup of the Week, 245–46

soups: Borscht, 244–45; Butternut Squash Soup with Ginger and Fennel, 246–47; Soup of the Week, 245–46

sour cream (Borscht), 244–45

spices. *See* herbs and spices

spinach: Chocolate, Cherry, and Spinach Shake, 232; Frittata, 234; Mushroom-Nut Pâté, 272; Smart Fat Shake, 229; Vanilla, Blueberry, and Spinach Shake, 231

squash: butternut, 246–47; yellow, 263; zucchini, 249–50, 262–63

Steak Kebobs with Pineapple, Onion, and Bell Pepper, 261–62

Stocks: Crab Cakes with Quinoa, 265–66; Moroccan Chicken Stew, 249–50. *See also* broths

Strawberries: Chocolate and Strawberry Shake, 232; Dark Chocolate Drizzle, 282–83

sweet potatoes (Soup of the Week), 245–46

Swiss Chard (Sautéed Swiss Chard with Garlic and Italian Herbs), 279

tamari sauce: Chicken Satay Skewers with Cabbage Wraps, 255–56; gluten-

tamari sauce *(continued)*
free, 255, 260; Marinated Flank Steak over Mixed Green Salad, 259–60
Tandoori Chicken, 253–54
temperature for cooking oil, 223, 224
thyme: Beef Stew, 262–63; Brussels Sprouts with Smart Lemon-Butter Sauce, 278–79; Chicken with Pecan-Herb Crust, 252; Crab Cakes with Quinoa, 265–66; keep supply of, 221; Mushroom-Nut Pâté, 272; Smart Vinaigrette Dressing, 243
tomatoes: Avocado, Cucumber, and Garbanzo Salad, 240; Beef Stew, 262–63; Borscht, 244–45; Frittata, 234; Marinated Flank Steak over Mixed Green Salad, 259–60; Moroccan Chicken Stew, 249–50; Shrimp, Fennel, and Cannellini Bean Salad with Orange Vinaigrette, 241–42; Sirloin Steak Chili, 258–59; Vegetable Korma, 274
Turkey Meatballs, 250–51

vacuum-packed frozen fish, 228
Vanilla, Blueberry, and Spinach Shake, 231
Vanilla, Cherry, and Kale Shake, 231
Vegetable Korma, 274
vegetables: Chicken Satay Skewers with Cabbage Wraps, 255–56; frozen, 227; keeping pantry supply of, 225–26; organic vs. not organic debate, 226. *See also specific vegetable*

vegetarian side dishes: Avocado, Cucumber, and Garbanzo Salad, 240; Borscht, 244; Butternut Squash Soup with Ginger and Fennel, 246; Frittata, 234; Lentil Curry, 273; Mushroom-Nut Pâté, 272; Omelet, 233; Raita, 275; Vegetable Korma, 274; White Bean Salad, 242; Wild Mushroom Soufflé, 275–76; Wild Rice and Quinoa with Kale and Almonds, 280
vinaigrette dressings: Shrimp, Fennel, and Cannellini Bean Salad with Orange Vinaigrette, 241–42; Smart Vinaigrette Dressing, 243

walnuts: Asian Pear, Gorgonzola Cheese, Walnuts, and Raspberries, 237; Broiled Oysters with Walnut, Parmesan Cheese, and Parsley Crust, 269; Fruit Salad with Mint, Lemon Rind, and Greek Yogurt, 283
White Bean Salad, 242–43
Wild Mushroom Soufflé, 275–76
Wild Rice and Quinoa with Kale and Slivered Almonds, 280–81

yogurt: Borscht, 244–45; Fruit Salad with Mint, Lemon Rind, and Greek Yogurt, 283; keeping pantry supply of, 225; Raita, 275; Tandoori Chicken, 253–54; Vegetable Korma, 274

zucchini: Beef Stew, 262–63; Moroccan Chicken Stew, 249–50

Subject Index

acetylcholine neurotransmitter, 43
acute inflammation, 18–19
ADD (attention deficit disorder), 154
adrenaline hormones, 206–7
adrenals, 206
agave nectar/syrup: high-fructose corn syrup (HFCS) in, 63–64
aging: free radical theory of, 41; and inflammation, 19–20; and Metabolic Syndrome, 77; and resveratrol, 194–95; and stress, 205; and sugar-coated proteins, 66
ALA (alpha linoleic acid), 185
alcoholic beverages: glycemic load (GL), 92; Phase 1, 111, 121; Phase 2, 126–27. *See also* beverages
allicin, 42
almond butter, 152
almond oil, 59
almonds: glycemic load (GL), 90; magnesium content, 179
Alzheimer's disease: and chronic inflammation, 19
American College of Nutrition, 38, 186
American Dietetic Association, 60, 73
American Heart Association, 60, 72, 76, 184
American Journal of Clinical Nutrition, 190
amygdala, 206
animal protein: 5-5-10 guidelines on eating clean, 98, 102–6; from grain-fed animals, 49–52; pasture-raised, 59

"animal vs. vegetable" debate, 3
anthocyanins, 38
antibiotics, 48–49
antioxidants, 38
appetite: and fiber, 35; and leptin, 25, 28–29, 30–31, 33, 85, 93, 210
apples: glycemic load (GL), 89; low-sugar fruit, 83
Aricept (donepezil), 43
artificial sweeteners: aspartame (NutraSweet and Equal), 144; comparing natural and artificial sweeteners, 62, 64, 143–44; saccharin, 144; sucralose (Splenda), 144. *See also* sugar
aspartame (NutraSweet and Equal), 144
Atkins Diet, 9–11
ATP (adenosine triphosphate), 178, 193
avocado glycemic load (GL), 91
avocado oil, 59

bakery products: glycemic load, 87
Barlean's, 172
basal metabolic rate (BMR), 164
bathroom scales: bioelectrical impedance (BEI), 162; pros and cons of regularly weighing yourself, 161–62
beans: 38, 39, 90, 108, 110, 115, 158–59, 179
beef: 49–50, 24; organic vs. nonorganic, 49
belly fat, 207–8. *See also* Metabolic Syndrome

berries: 83; glycemic load (GL), 90
beta-carotene, 38
beverages: fruit juice, 63–64, 82, 83, 84, 88, 137–38. *See also* alcoholic beverages; hydration
bioelectrical impedance (BEI) scale, 162
biotin (vitamin B$_7$), 177
bitter taste, 158
blood pressure: and fiber, 35; and Metabolic Syndrome, 77
blood sugar levels: and citrus bergamot, 195; and sugary foods, 60. *See also* insulin
blueberries: glycemic load (GL), 89
body fat level, 106, 162
boron, 177
brain: Alzheimer's disease, 12, 19; memory loss, 19, 44–45; exercise, 198–200; stress, 206
brain fog, 19
breakfast: Phase 1, 121–25; Phase 2, 127–35; Smart Fat Shake for, 105, 115, 116–18; recommendations for, 115
Broussard, J. L., 211
Buettner, Dan, 215
butter, 24, 53, 59

calcium: controversy, 180–81; relationship with magnesium, 179
calories: and exercise, 203
Campylobacter, 145
cancer: and chronic inflammation, 19
canola oil, 59
cantaloupe, 83
carbohydrates: 60, 61–62, 70–75, 85–86, 87, 88, 89, 92, 153; "Dietary Goals for the United States" recommendations, 70; and fiber-rich foods, 37; and glycemic load, 84–85; starchy, 11, 12, 72–73. *See also* macronutrients; refined carbohydrates
cardamom, 42, 44
carotenoids, 177
celiac disease, 61
Centers for Disease Control and Prevention, 65, 105
CGMP (current good manufacturing practices), 173

cheese, 24, 53
cherries, 83
chia seeds: and fiber, 109; and omega-3, 185
chips: glycemic load, 89; healthy substitutes, 150
cholesterol: and citrus bergamot, 195; and coconut oil, 101; and eggs 140–41; and fiber 38; LDL (low-density lipoprotein), 23, 44, 54, 56, 77–78, 101
chromium, 177
chronic inflammation, 19–20
cinnamon, 44
circadian rhythms, 209–10
citrus bergamot, 195
Clean Fifteen list, 156–57. *See also* Environmental Working Group
clean protein: description of, 13–14, vs. "mean" protein, 15; guidelines on eating, 98, 102–6. *See also* mean protein; protein
cocoa: flavanols, 151; powder, 109
coconut, 23
coconut oil, 23, 59, 91, 101
coenzyme Q10 (or CoQ10), 192–94
coffee, 88, 145–46, 151
cognitive decline: and chronic inflammation, 19; and exercise, 198–200; and memory loss, 19, 44–45
copper, 177
corn oil, 59
cortisol, 25, 31–33, 85, 206–8, 212, 214
crackers, 89
cream, 24
cumin, 42
curcumin, 164, 191–92
cytokines, 20

dairy foods: and smart fat, 52–53; and glycemic load (GL), 89; and pesticides and chemical contamination, 49
dark chocolate: and fiber, 109, 110, 115; and glycemic load (GL), 89; and smart fat, 23, 115
deep breathing practice, 208–9
detox supplements, 164–65
DHA (docosahexaenoic acid), 56, 171, 184–85

diabetes: 12; and high-fructose corn syrup (HFCS), 63; and omega–3 fatty acids, 184; and vitamin D deficiency, 186

diets: Atkins Diet, 9–11; fads and failures, 68–70; Mediterranean, 159; Pritikin Diet, 10, 11; Standard American Diet (SAD), 11–12

diet soda, 143

dinner meal plans: Phase 1, 121–25; Phase 2, 127–35

dioxins, 47–48

Dirty Dozen list, 156. *See also* Environmental Working Group

"dirty" oils: definition, 55–56; health effects, 56–57

disease: and chronic inflammation, 19–20; and omega–6 to omega–3 ratio, 22, 47, 56; psychoneuroimmunology, 217; and refined carbohydrates, 60–61; and Standard American Diet (SAD), 12

EGCG (epigallocatechin gallate), 121, 188–91. *See also* green tea

eggs: and cholesterol, 140–41; guidelines on eating, 98, 102–6; glycemic load (GL), 91; omega–3 fatty acids, 53; as smart fat and protein source, 115

emotional intelligence, 216–17

Environmental Working Group (EWG): Clean Fifteen, 156–57; Dirty Dozen, 156

EPA (eicosapentaenoic acid), 56, 171, 184–85

Epsom salts, 178

erythritol, 144, 145

estrogen, 33, 34

exercise: 74–75, 146–47, 198–204; weight training, 202–3

extra-virgin olive oil, 59

fast food diet, 75

fat burning: and inflammation, 20

fats, 2, 22–24, 65, 66. *See also* macronutrients; smart fats

FDA (Food and Drug Administration), 57, 173

fiber, 36–39, 98, 107–11

fish: and fish oil, 23, 115, 171, 179, 183–4. *See also* oils

flavor, 15, 40–41. *See also* spices

flax seeds, 23, 185

folic acid (folates), 177

Food and Nutrition Board (Institute of Medicine), 102

food diary, 160–61

food guide pyramid (USDA), 82

food labels: and sugar, 62; and trans fats, 58

food preparation: and glycemic load (GL), 92

food sources: dumb fats, 23–24; high in fiber, 39; neutral fats, 24; refined carbohydrates, 61–62; smart fat, 23

free radical theory of aging, 41

free-range USDA guidelines, 53

fruit juice, 63–64, 82, 83, 84, 88, 137–38

Garden of Life, 172

garlic, 42–43

genetically modified organisms (GMOs), 41

glycemic index, 84; vs. glycemic load (GL), 85–86

glycemic load (GL), 11, 84–93

GMOS. *See* genetically modified organisms

good fats. *See* smart fats

grain-based foods: 5–5–10 guidelines on fiber through, 108–9; glycemic load (GL), 88–89; high glycemic load (GL) of all, 93

grain-fed animals: eating clean protein instead of, 50–52; negative health effects of, 49–50

green light oils, 59

green tea (EGCG, epigallocatechin gallate), 121, 188–91

growth hormones, 48

hazelnuts, 23, 90

HDL cholesterol: and citrus bergamot, 195; and coconut oil, 101; and eggs, 140; and Metabolic Syndrome, 77–78; and triglycerides, 78

heart disease: 12; and Seven Countries
    Study, 71–73; and chronic inflamma-
    tion, 19; and high-fructose corn syrup
    (HFCS), 63; and Metabolic Syndrome
    (prediabetes), 56, 76, 184
herbs: 15, 41–42, 43–44; as antioxi-
    dants, 41
high blood sugar levels, 77
high fasting blood sugar, 77
high-fructose corn syrup (HFCS),
    63–64, 74
high-sensitivity C-reactive protein
    (hs CRP), 19
HIIT (high-intensity interval training),
    201–2, 204
hormones: cortisol, 25, 31–33, 85, 206–8,
    212, 214; growth hormones, 48; human
    growth hormone (HGH), 212; insulin,
    25–28, 35, 84–85, 211; leptin, 25,
    28–29, 28–31, 30–31, 33, 85, 93, 210;
    melatonin, 212; sex hormones, 33–34;
    and smart fats, 25–33
human growth hormone, 212
hydration, 127, 162, 165. *See also* beverages
hydrogenated oils, 23, 54, 58, 74. *See also*
    trans fats

immune system: and inflammation,
    18–20, 217. *See also* psychoneuroim-
    munology
inflammation: acute, 18–19; chronic,
    19–20; description and function
    in the body, 18; and fiber, 35; and
    Metabolic Syndrome, 77; and
    omega–3 fatty, 22, 184. *See also*
    anti-inflammatory foods; omega–6
    fatty acids
insoluble fiber, 35
insulin: 25–28; and glycemic load,
    84–85; and fiber, 35; and sleep, 211.
    See also blood sugar levels; sugar
insulin resistance, 60, 78, 186, 194, 211;
    and cortisol levels, 207; and high-
    fructose corn syrup (HFCS), 63; and
    stress, 78, 207
insulin sensitivity, 79, 155, 183, 186,
    189, 211
interval training exercise, 201–2, 204

juicing, 138–40

Keys, Ancel, 71–72, 73, 140. *See also*
    Seven Countries Study

lactase enzyme, 153–54
lactose intolerant, 153–54, 155
lard, 24, 59
LDL (low-density lipoprotein), 23, 44, 54,
    56, 77–78, 140
leafy green vegetables: and magnesium,
    179; and vitamin K, 182
lean protein, 52–53
lectins, 158–59
legumes, 1, 39, 91, 108, 115; and
    magnesium, 179
leptin, 25, 28–29, 30–31, 33, 83, 85, 93,
    112, 119, 210
linoleic acid, 56
lunch meal plans: Phase 1, 121–25;
    Phase 2, 127–35

macadamia nuts, 23, 59, 91
macronutrients, 73. *See also*
    carbohydrates; fats; proteins
magnesium: 11, 179; and calcium, 179;
    and smart fat, 177–78; supplements,
    172, 179
Masley Optimal Health Center,
    186, 199
MCT (medium-chain triglyceride) oil,
    23, 116, 117
meal plans: Phase 1, 121–25; Phase 2,
    127–35
mean protein: vs. clean protein, 15;
    health consequences, 15. *See also*
    clean protein
Mediterranean eating plan, 159
memory loss: and chronic
    inflammation, 19; and turmeric,
    44–45
Metabolic Syndrome: prediabetes,
    76–79; and citrus bergamot, 195; and
    high-fructose corn syrup (HFCS), 63;
    and omega–3 fatty acids, 184. *See also*
    belly fat; weight gain
metabolism: basal metabolic
    rate (BMR), 164; and protein,

39–40; and green tea and EGCG (epigallocatechin gallate), 188–91

micronutrients, 173

milk: 24, 53, 88, 145–46, 153–54, 155; organic, 146; raw, 145

milk thistle, 164

mitochondria, 20

multivitamins, 170–72, 175–77, 186

NAFLD (nonalcoholic fatty-liver disease), 56

NASH (nonalcoholic steatohepatitis), 56

natural sweeteners: vs. artificial, 62, 64, 143–44; erythritol, 144, 145; stevia, 144, 145; xylitol, 144, 145. *See also* sugar

neutral fats, 24, 47–50, 54–57

nut oils, 59, 91

nuts: and fiber, 39, 110, 115; and glycemic load (GL), 90–91; and magnesium, 179; and smart fat, 23, 115

obesity: 12, 21, 24, 58–59, 61–62, 69, 72–73; and diet soda, 143; and inflammation, 19

oils: hydrogenated and partially hydrogenated, 23, 54, 58–59, 74; MCT (medium-chain triglyceride) oil, 23, 116, 117. *See also* omega–3 fatty acids

olive oil: 23, 59; extra-virgin vs. regular, 59

olives: glycemic load (GL), 91; as smart fat source, 23

omega–3 fatty acids: DHA (docosahexaenoic acid): 56, 171, 184–85; EPA (eicosapentaenoic acid), 56, 171, 184–85; fish oil, 171, 183–85; and inflammation, 22, 184; and eggs, 53

omega–6 fatty acids: 24, 54–57; pro-inflammatory properties, 21–22. *See also* inflammation

omega–6 to omega–3 ratio, 22, 47, 49, 56

orange juice, 137–38

oranges, 83, 137–38

organic food: beef, 49; butter, 59; milk, 146, 156–57

oxidation: and beans, 38; and herbs and spices, 41

OXLAMS (oxidized linoleic acid metabolites), 56

partially hydrogenated oils, 23, 54, 57, 74. *See also* trans fats

pasta, 85–86, 89, 92, 152

pasture-raised cows, 59

pasture-raised ducks, 59

peaches, 83, 90

peanut butter, 151–52

peanuts, 91

pears, 83, 90

peanut oil, 59

pecan oil, 59

pecans, 23, 91

pesticides, 47–48, 156

Phase 1, alcohol and food restrictions, 111, 121; meal plans, 121–25

Phase 2, 111–14, 126–35

pistachio oil, 59

pistachios, 23, 91

polyphenols, 188, 189

polyunsaturated fats: omega–6 fatty acids, 21–22; "saturated vs. unsaturated" debate, 3

potassium, 11, 157–58

prediabetes. *See* Metabolic Syndrome

Pritikin Diet, 10–11

probiotics, 187–88

processed foods, 11, 12

progesterone, 33, 34

protein: 13–15, 49–52, 59, 91, 106; and sugar, 65–66. *See also* clean protein; macronutrients

protein bars, 150–51

psychoneuroimmunology, 217

RDAs (recommended daily allowances), 170–71

red light oils, 59

red palm oil, 59

refined carbohydrates: 60–61; cupcakes, 65–67; foods made with flour, 61–62; foods with added sugar, 62–65; increased consumption, 75. *See also* carbohydrates

REM sleep, 212, 213
resveratrol (trans-resveratrol), 194–95

saccharin, 144
sage, 42, 43
salty foods, 157–58
saturated fats: 24; "saturated vs.
    unsaturated" debate, 3
sedentary lifestyle, 74–75
seeds, 23, 39, 115, 179
selenium, 164–65, 177
sesame oil, 59
Seven Countries Study, 71–73
sex hormones: estrogen, 33, 34;
    progesterone, 33, 34; testosterone,
    33–34
sleep: circadian rhythms and, 209–10;
    importance of getting adequate, 209,
    210; improving, 214–15; and insulin
    levels, 211; sleep architecture, 212–14;
    and weight gain, 210–12
sleep architecture: non-REM sleep,
    212–13; REM sleep, 212, 213
smart fats: 2–3, 13, 17–23, 25–33, 52–53,
    57–59, 112–15; guidelines on, 98,
    99–101, 112
Smart Fat Shake, 105, 115, 116–18
Smart Fat Solution components: fiber,
    15; flavor, 15; protein, 13–15; smart
    fat, 13
smoking, 74
soda: artificial sweeteners and diet, 143;
    glycemic load (GL), 88
sodium, 157
soluble fiber, 35
soybean oil, 59
spaghetti: glycemic index, 85–86;
    glycemic load (GL), 89, 92
spices: health properties of, 15; 41–42; as
    antioxidants, 41; savory, 44–45. *See
    also* flavor
sports drinks, 64
Standard American Diet (SAD):
    description, 11–12; detoxing from,
    164–65; and fiber, 187
starchy carbohydrates: and obesity,
    72–73; and Standard American Diet
    (SAD), 11, 12

steel-cut oats, 88, 141, 142–43
stevia, 144, 145
stress, 204–9
stress hormones (cortisol), 25, 31–33, 85,
    206–8, 212, 214
sucralose (Splenda), 144
sugar: and obesity, 72–73; added to foods,
    62–65; high-fructose corn syrup
    (HFCS), 63–64, 74; sugar-fat combo,
    65, 66; sugar-protein combo, 65–66.
    See also artificial sweeteners; insulin
supplements: citrus bergamot, 195;
    coenzyme Q10 (or CoQ10), 192–94;
    curcumin, 164, 191–92; DHA
    (docosahexaenoic acid), 56, 171,
    184–85; EGCG (epigallocatechin
    gallate) [green tea extract], 121,
    188–91; EPA (eicosapentaenoic acid),
    56, 171, 184–85; fish oil, 171, 183–85;
    magnesium, 172, 179; milk thistle,
    164; *N*-acetylcysteine (NAC), 164;
    PaleoFiber, 109; probiotics, 187–88;
    recommendations, 174–75, 196;
    resveratrol (trans-resveratrol), 194–
    95; selenium, 164–65; Sunfiber, 109;
    vitamin C, 192; vitamin D, 185–87;
    vitamin K, 183

testosterone, 33–34
Therapeutic Goods Administration
    (TGA) standards [Australia], 174
toxins, 47–52
trans fats, 23, 54, 57–58, 74, 75
trans-resveratrol (resveratrol), 194–95
triglycerides: and citrus bergamot, 195;
    and high-fructose corn syrup (HFCS),
    63–64; and Metabolic Syndrome, 77;
    ratio to HDL cholesterol, 78; and fish
    oil, 183–84
turmeric, 44–45
25-hydroxy vitamin D test, 186

umani, 158
USDA: Certified Organic label, 53; food
    guide pyramid, 82

"vegetable oil blend," 59
vegetable oils, 21, 24, 58

vegetables: 107–8, 110; glycemic load, 91, 93; and magnesium 179

vitamin A, 177

vitamin B$_1$ (thiamin), 177

vitamin B$_2$ (riboflavin), 177

vitamin B$_3$ (niacin), 177

vitamin B$_5$, 177

vitamin B$_6$ (pyridoxine), 177

vitamin B$_7$ (biotin), 177

vitamin B$_{12}$, 177

vitamin C, 170, 177, 192

vitamin D: 170; reco, 177; 185–87

vitamin D2 (ergocalciferol), 187

vitamin D3 (cholecalciferol), 187

vitamin E, 177

vitamin K, 177, 182–83

walking, 201–2

walnut oil, 59

walnuts, 23, 91

weight gain: and sleep deficiency, 210–12; self-monitoring, 161–62.

See also Metabolic Syndrome

weight loss: and clean protein, 39–40; and eating fat, 2, 159–60; and green tea and EGCG, 189–91; and chronic inflammation, 20; and fiber, 36, 38; and vitamin D, 186

weight-loss plateau: 163–65; and inflammation, 20

weight training, 202–3

white flour, 61–62

whole-grain flour: 79–82; 141; vs. white flour, 62; glycemic load (GL), 87

wine. *See* alcoholic beverages

xylitol, 144, 145

yellow light oils, 59

yogurt: 24, 53; glycemic load (GL), 89; homemade, 146

zinc, 177